The Clinical Medical
Librarian's Handbook

Medical Library Association Books

The Medical Library Association (MLA) publishes state-of-the-art books that enhance health care, support professional development, improve library services, and promote research throughout the world.

MLA books are dynamic resources for librarians in hospitals, medical research practice, corporate libraries, and other settings. These invaluable publications provide medical librarians, health-care professionals, and patients with accurate information that can improve outcomes and save lives.

The MLA Books Panel is responsible for (1) monitoring publishing trends within the industry, (2) exploring new concepts in publications by actively soliciting and proposing ideas for new publications, and (3) coordinating publishing efforts to achieve the best utilization of MLA resources. Each MLA book is directly administered from its inception by the MLA Books Panel, composed of MLA members with expertise spanning the breadth of health sciences librarianship.

Medical Library Association Books Panel

About the Medical Library Association

The Medical Library Association is a global, nonprofit, educational organization with a membership of more than 400 institutions and 3,000 professionals in the health information field. Since 1898, MLA has fostered excellence in the professional practice and leadership of health sciences library and information professionals to enhance health care, education, and research throughout the world. MLA educates health information professionals, supports health information research, promotes access to the world's health sciences information, and works to ensure that the best health information is available to all.

Books in the Series

The Clinical Medical Librarian's Handbook

Edited by
Judy C. Stribling

ROWMAN & LITTLEFIELD
Lanham • Boulder • New York • London

Published by Rowman & Littlefield
An imprint of The Rowman & Littlefield Publishing Group, Inc.
4501 Forbes Boulevard, Suite 200, Lanham, Maryland 20706
www.rowman.com

6 Tinworth Street, London SE11 5AL

British Library Cataloguing in Publication Information Available

Library of Congress Cataloging-in-Publication Data

Names: Stribling, Judy C., 1961– editor.
Title: The clinical medical librarian's handbook / edited by Judy C. Stribling.
Description: Lanham, Maryland : Rowman & Littlefield, [2020] | Series: Medical Library Associa-
    tion books | Includes bibliographical references and index. | Summary: "With contributions by
    experts working in academic medical centers, Clinical Medical Librarianship provides descrip-
    tions of innovative initiatives and programs such as a curriculum for teaching the next generation
    of medical librarians, recognizing the importance of patient-centered care, and strengthening
    relationships with clinicians"—Provided by publisher.
Identifiers: LCCN 2019038976 (print) | LCCN 2019038977 (ebook) | ISBN 9781538127704 (paper-
    back) | ISBN 9781538127711 (epub)
Subjects: LCSH: Medical librarianship—United States. | Medical librarians—Professional relation-
    ships—United States. | Medical libraries—United States—Case studies.
Classification: LCC Z675.M4 .C595 2020 (print) | LCC Z675.M4 (ebook) | DDC 026/.61—dc23
LC record available at https://lccn.loc.gov/2019038976
LC ebook record available at https://lccn.loc.gov/2019038977

Contents

List of Tables

List of Figures

Foreword

I was first introduced to clinical medical librarians through the New York Academy of Medicine evidence-based medicine (EBM) course in 2007. As a junior faculty, I led "Journal Club," where pediatric residents used EBM principles to analyze manuscripts and determine the applicability to their clinical question. I attended this course to learn about EBM; however, I was introduced to clinical medical librarians in their role as *course leader*. As I sat through classes, I could not help but think what an amazing resource a clinical librarian is and all the wonderful ways in which we could collaborate to improve care for our patients.

The timing was right: in 2006 at our departmental strategic retreat, several initiatives were mapped out as our future direction, including the implementation of patient- and family-centered care, further development of our patient safety and quality programs, and programs to improve our patients' perception of care. At the same time, the clinical medical librarians at our institution aimed to develop and grow their activities.

We were very fortunate to have the opportunity to work with Judy Stribling and her colleagues from the beginning of this joint journey. Judy is an amazing and knowledgeable resource with a vision, persistence, and passion that can only lead to success.

We began by inviting clinical medical librarians to participate in family-centered rounds. During family-centered rounds (FCRs), families are invited to participate in clinical decisions along with the medical team, including physicians, mid-level providers, nurses, students, and other support staff. The care discussions and education on these rounds allows for many opportunities to seek librarians' input in the format of EBM questions. For example, on rounds we could be addressing a case of a baby with a fever with an acute urinary tract infection, and because current American Academy of Pediatrics guidelines are written for infants and children two months to two years of age, we may not have information on the optimal length of antibiotic therapy. Clinical librarians would help us address this question by accessing the appropriate literature, interacting with our trainees, and teaching EBM at the point of care.

The librarian may stay behind or return to a family after the medical team has moved to the next patient to provide further patient/family-centered education. For example, a family of a child with a new diagnosis may have additional questions about the diagnosis or treatment plan that were not shared with the medical team during rounds. However, upon hearing that a medical librarian is on the team, the family may engage with them to provide further support knowing that they are a trusted information source who can locate information without medical jargon and at the appropriate level of health literacy.

Even though we have a wonderful patient education center across the street from the hospital where children are cared for, families are unlikely to leave the bedside of their children. Instead, we established regular "library hours" adjacent to our patient care units. Families are encouraged to come during these hours and have their questions answered by a library expert.

You can only imagine what this can do for patient satisfaction and their overall feeling about support during their hospital stay.

Likewise, our faculty and trainees have access to clinical medical librarians when conducting research. This can be in a form of literature review, specifically if we need to access databases with which we may not be familiar. This is also helpful when we are developing educational tools and need to make sure that our material is at the appropriate health literacy level, or when we are engaged in patient-centered outcomes research and we need to determine how to best engage our patients in research.

As I have grown in my academic and professional roles from junior to senior faculty, from medical director of the General Pediatric Unit to vice chair for quality and patient safety, so have the many roles and activities of our clinical medical librarians. It is evident that we (I) could not do this job well without input from our librarians. They have become integral members of our teams. We celebrate our librarians at every turn in our daily activities.

This comprehensive handbook will provide you with information and tools that you will be able to use to develop the program that will best suit your needs. Without a doubt, your patients will get medical information that they need at the level and in the format that they can make the best use of. Likewise, your trainees and faculty will thank you for enabling their education and scholarly activity.

Dr. Snezana Nena Osorio

Preface

Sharing the blended knowledge and experience of medical librarians who developed innovative and successful programs in their libraries and hospitals with other librarians is the main goal of this book. Each contributor to this text—from library director to consumer health librarian—practices in a major urban academic medical center and engages in educating their community's population about new technologies and the importance of providing evidence-based and literacy-level-appropriate information to every individual participant in health-care settings. The authors wrote this book because they realized the breadth and reach of a Medical Library Association publication could encourage other librarians to explore similar programs.

Discovering what characterizes strong clinical medical librarianship and how those characteristics have been and are supporting clinicians in their delivery of evidence-based medicine (EBM) can help librarians evaluate and strengthen their own programs. Perhaps more importantly, learning from leaders in clinical medical librarianship can help other librarians provide clinicians and other health-care professionals with strategies to ensure that their programs stay abreast of the rapidly changing health-care field using methods and approaches that adapt to new technology and research requirements.

The Clinical Medical Librarian's Handbook details the history of clinical medical librarianship and provides a series of vignettes and case studies that illustrate ways medical librarians continue to advance the field by creating valuable services for patients and caregivers and providing innovative learning experiences for clinicians, medical and library students, and practicing medical librarians.

ORGANIZATION AND CONTENT

The Clinical Medical Librarian's Handbook piques readers' interest by describing historical overviews and sharing innovative programs. Keith C. Mages and Terrie R. Wheeler open the text with a chapter that traces the initial services of Gertrude Lamb and her team to the evolution of the modern clinical medical librarian (CML). Chapter 1 informs the following chapters that explore the expanding role of the CML.

Authors Judy C. Stribling and Antonio P. DeRosa discuss the advantages of creating strong partnerships with clinicians. While recognizing the challenges in building these relationships, Stribling and DeRosa suggest strategies for developing and maintaining them by stepping out of the library, engaging in as many campus-wide events as possible, and remaining in step with their clinical customers.

DeRosa and Becky Baltich Nelson discuss the emergence and importance of patient- and family-centered care (PFCC). The authors explore the history of PFCC and the implications the practice has on changing the landscape of the U.S. health-care system. In chapters 4 and 5, Stribling and DeRosa continue the discussion of PFCC and describe two unique programs developed at their institution.

Timothy Roberts explains the role of the librarian in public health. Health librarians are challenged to develop new skills and expertise in accessing different types of information to meet the needs of public health researchers. Roberts points out the intertwining concepts of public health and ways librarians can provide support for expert informatics systems.

WCM librarians describe fun and entertaining methods used by librarians at WCM to highlight their library resources and new technologies. Curating curriculum-specific resources, making the most of the competitive nature of medical students, and hosting a campus-wide technology fair are some of the ways WCM librarians expose their community members to tools to enable lifelong learning and appreciate the library.

Demonstrating the value of CML roles to an institution is challenging. Marisol Hernandez maps one hospital's journey to magnet and discusses the impact librarians have on the success of this significant and costly undertaking. Positively affecting the financial bottom line of an institution is a unique opportunity for librarians to demonstrate their value and raise the profile of the library.

Rachel Pinotti acknowledges the importance of the CML role in teaching evidence-based medicine to students and discusses some of the common challenges faced by instructors and learners. Pinotti suggests ways CMLs can leverage their EBM role to become more involved in medical education curriculums.

Mages and Baltich Nelson recognize the difficulty a new librarian faces when trying to break into practice in a clinical medical setting. A CML internship program that provides intensive on-the-job training for new librarians is described.

Library director Terrie R. Wheeler's concluding chapter provides encouragement to other library administrators who wish to transform their clinical programs. Wheeler's use of a logic model to develop and execute administrative initiatives offers an almost step-by-step methodology for creating and managing change.

The underlying message of *The Clinical Medical Librarian's Handbook* demonstrates the ability of CMLs to continually evolve and remain valuable partners to clinicians, students, and institutions. CMLs improve and enhance patient care and clinical decision-making.

AUDIENCE AND APPLICATION

The Clinical Medical Librarian's Handbook is intended for any library student, practicing librarian, or health administrator interested in understanding the variety of roles medical librarians play in the health-care system of the United States, how medical librarians interact with clinicians and patients, the power of patient-centered care and technology, the importance of information to public health, novel ways to introduce and teach clinical learners to use resources, how clinical medical librarians learn to do the job, and tips for managing clinical medical library programs.

Chapter One

An Introduction to Hospitals, Research, and Medical Libraries

Keith C. Mages and Terrie R. Wheeler

I went out as a member of the patient care team, along with the clinical pharmacist and the clinical dietitian and the social worker and the physician . . . and I discovered that all of those team members had information needs that were never met. [1]—Gertrude Lamb, March 31, 1985

When Gertrude Lamb first stepped onto the general medicine ward of the Kansas City General Hospital and Medical Center in 1971, professional innovation was not her goal. Lamb arrived at the teaching hospital of the University of Missouri–Kansas City (UMKC) with the intention of aligning the library's services with the evolving needs of UMKC's new medical school curriculum. Lamb conducted an information needs assessment that included observing the daily educational environment of UMKC medical students, faculty, and hospital staff on clinical rounds. [2] Lamb realized students and clinicians posed questions during clinical rounds that were often unanswered. Inspiration struck, and the clinical medical librarianship role was born.

Examination of mid-twentieth-century American medicine, hospitals, and medical libraries frames discussion of the history of clinical medical librarianship programs. The practice of medicine and medical technology evolved rapidly during World War II and the following years. Likewise, the body of published medical literature increased. A substantial boost to the National Institutes of Health funding accounts for some of the increase in publications. [3] Federal funding programs designed to increase the numbers of American health-care professionals, such as the Health Professions Educational Assistance Act of 1963 and the Nurse Training Act of 1964, were also factors.

1

MEDICAL LIBRARY ASSISTANCE ACT OF 1965

Several federal initiatives influenced medical libraries during the 1960s. Proposals from 1962's *Surgeon General's Conference on Health Communications* formed the backbone of the Medical Library Assistance Act. Aimed to improve transfer of information from scientists to health-care workers and on to the public, the conference proposal suggested that biomedical libraries serve as centers of communication and receive additional federal funding for exploration of new roles and technologies.[4] The 1965 *Report of the President's Commission on Heart Disease, Cancer and Stroke* called for increased dissemination of health-care research, particularly around burgeoning chronic diseases; the *Commission* also transferred oversight of extramural support programs from the Public Health Service to the National Library of Medicine (NLM).[5]

The proposal and report informed the Medical Library Assistance Act (MLAA) of 1965, which funded health sciences libraries to create more effective services and resources to meet evolving needs. Specifically, the MLAA sought to establish the NLM as the locus for nation-wide biomedical library development. Funds enabled the NLM to provide grants to the library community for the following activities:

- Constructing new or renovating existing biomedical libraries
- Educating and training medical librarians and other health information specialists
- Assisting researchers on special scientific projects
- Researching projects in the field of medical librarianship
- Building biomedical library collections and exploring new technology
- Establishing a national network of regional medical libraries (RML)
- Preparing biomedical scientific publications[6]

The national network of RMLs created a unique model for dissemination of biomedical research. The RML network established health sciences libraries in eleven (later trimmed to seven) geographic locations as regional biomedical communications hubs. The RMLs supported their regions by awarding grants to smaller libraries for training librarians and health professionals on NLM resources and marketing the RMLs' role in biomedical communications.[7]

JOINT COMMISSION AND HOSPITAL LIBRARY STANDARDS

Two years later, the Joint Commission on Accreditation of Hospitals (JCAH), now known as the Joint Commission, established the Medical Library Advisory Committee. Tasked to identify and define hospital library standards, this committee—composed of five librarians, three physicians, and one hospital administrator—recommended staffing at least one full-time librarian to provide adequate and accessible library collections, reference, document delivery, and audiovisual services to hospitals.[8]

LATCH PROGRAMS

In 1967, the NLM funded librarian Jane Fulcher's Literature ATtached to CHarts (LATCH) program.[9] LATCH programming assumed patients would receive better care if their clinicians were aware of the most current developments in medicine. LATCH introduced the practice of providing rapid and patient-specific literature to clinicians on the wards. Initially, Washington Hospital librarians followed predetermined guidelines—developed by medical department heads and members of hospital administration—to identify patients for LATCH services. Clinicians received information packets, or "LATCHes," focusing on the pathophysiology of a patient's admitting condition. However, admitting diagnoses evolved over the course of hospitalization and rendered original LATCHes less relevant and helpful. Even if a patient's diagnosis remained stable, librarians noticed physicians were not interested in the generalized, review-type literature contained in LATCHes.[10]

In light of this, librarians revised the process and made extensive changes to LATCH at the beginning of 1968. Instead of attaching general literature based on admitting diagnoses, librarians worked with clinicians to identify particularly vexing or unusual patient cases. Under the new system, literature requested by clinical staff addressed specific questions, and information provided in LATCHes was more relevant to the patient's treatment plan. Hence, LATCH evolved into an "ordered" service, similar to diagnostic tests, drugs, and other aspects of hospital care.

Creators of LATCH assumed attending physicians and nurses would be the heaviest users of the service but discovered interns and residents requested more LATCHes than any other group. This highlighted the educational value of the program, and the grant rolled into a full-service program. A second librarian joined the team, workflow changed, and productivity increased to ensure delivery of LATCHes to clinicians within two hours of request.[11] LATCH librarians developed professional expertise and observed the most current developments in clinical medicine, controversies, and trends.

Following the success at Washington Hospital Center, institutions in Minneapolis and Boston initiated similar LATCH programs.[12] In 1982, Pennsylvania's Lehigh Valley Hospital Center computerized LATCH requests through the hospital's information system. Physicians and staff initiated LATCH requests directly from the patient's electronic medical record.[13]

GERTRUDE LAMB AND THE
CLINICAL MEDICAL LIBRARIAN MOVEMENT

Gertrude Lamb (1918–2015) widely considered the pioneering force of the clinical medical librarian movement, earned a bachelor's degree in economics from Radcliffe College (1940) and a master's degree in public administration from Boston University (1945). After teaching government and international relations at the University of Connecticut, Lamb enrolled in a master's of library science program at Case Western Reserve University. Upon completion of this program in 1968, Lamb continued at Case and pursued a doctoral education in information science and earned her Ph.D. in 1971.[14]

That same year Lamb accepted a position as medical librarian and associate professor of medicine at the University of Missouri–Kansas City. Here Lamb conceptualized and established the first clinical librarian program. In a 1985 oral history, Lamb recalled she never intended to initiate a novel professional role for librarians.[15] Indeed, she signed on to align medical library initiatives with the UMKC School of Medicine's newly designed academic plan, centered on a docent system of instruction.[16] In this context, a "docent" is a UMKC clinician-scholar responsible for the education of a subset of medical students. Each docent team consisted of a "senior docent, three docents, sabbatical leave physicians, residents, interns, nurses, pharmacists, ancillary personnel and the team of students."[17] Medical students received the bulk of their education and training in the patient-care setting, on rounds facilitated by the docent teams. In this novel system of tutor-based education, students learned anatomic and physiologic principles as well as proper diagnosis and treatment in the context of their assigned patient's disease states.[18]

Lamb joined the docent teams on the floors of UMKC's teaching hospital, Kansas City General Hospital, known today as Truman Medical Center, to assess her constituents' needs.[19] Rounding at the patient bedside with the multidisciplinary team introduced Lamb to a realm of collaboration in which each member had a specific role and duty. Docent team members often discussed information they wished was available or professed a lack of knowledge on a specific topic, but moved on without acquiring answers to explicit or implicit information needs. Based on these observations, Lamb identified a role for information specialists who could "go back and bring (the information) to the team very quickly so it was still in the context of the patient that they saw."[20]

Galvanized by her discovery, Lamb submitted a Public Health Service Grant application, titled "Biomedical Librarians in the Patient Care Setting," to NLM. Lamb asked for funds to "plan and evaluate a program to meet the biomedical communication needs of medical students, house officers, physicians, and health care team members in a representative general hospital."[21] Lamb's skillful wording linked the information role to the interdisciplinary clinical teams. The NLM funded Lamb to hire three science information specialists. This title was soon changed to clinical medical librarian (CML), to identify the professional and typical practice environment more accurately.[22] By August 1972, Lamb had hired three CMLs with library science degrees and training or education in medical librarianship. Each CML served a specific docent team to foster close connections within assigned clinical groups.

LIBRARIANS ON THE WARD AT UNIVERSITY OF MISSOURI–KANSAS CITY

At UMKC, a CML's typical day consisted of attending morning teaching rounds followed by time answering direct and anticipated questions. Each CML completed an average of eighty to one hundred MEDLINE searches per month and reported an average time of 7.2 minutes per search.[23] CMLs delivered results to their docent teams using a variety of information techniques. One CML adopted the LATCH system, attaching clinically relevant literature directly to the patient's chart, along with a bibliography of additional citations for those interested in studying the pathological process or medical technique in depth. Another developed a weekly publication titled *Current References* that combined an editorial, abstracts, and historic article based on specific patient needs. The third CML created a system called *Latest Topics* that included literature related to anticipated team needs in addition to specific requests.

Life on the wards could be difficult for those in these new roles. In her oral history, Lamb noted the CML role demanded a certain type of personality; CMLs must be "bright," "curious," with a "strong service orientation and . . . a pretty sturdy ego."[24] Lamb coined the term *brutal friendliness* to refer to a style of interaction she witnessed on the hospital floors. Lamb cautioned that CMLs must be prepared to participate in starkly direct communication on docent teams where friendly banter, sharp critique, and quick rebuttals were commonplace.[25] CMLs also needed to be prepared for initial underutilization and role misunderstanding. According to Lamb, respect would eventually develop, typically after a CML successfully searched, screened, and delivered literature based on perceived questions to the docent teams only hours after morning rounds.[26]

An Interview from the Field

Carolyn Reid was the first clinical medical librarian hired by Gertrude Lamb at UMKC. She began her role in September of 1971. A graduate of the University of Missouri–Columbia School of Library and Information Science, Reid's undergraduate degree is in speech and theater. After nine years at UMKC, Reid was hired as online services coordinator and later associate director at the Midcontinental Regional Medical Library Program at the University of Nebraska Medical Center in Omaha. Then, in 1987, she moved to Cornell University Medical College (now Weill Cornell Medical College), first as associate director (1987–2001) and then as director (2001–2010). She currently resides in New York City with her husband, Mark Funk (who was also an early CML at UMKC).

KM: Can you talk a little bit regarding what drew you to investigate this opportunity [with Gertrude Lamb, in clinical medical librarianship]?
CR: Well . . . I needed a job, and this one, originally titled science information specialist, sounded much more interesting than a traditional reference job. The other two interviews I had done were for reference positions, which was my main interest. This sounded very interesting because of the medical school: it was a new school, everything was new and different, and nobody knew exactly what they were doing. Like I said, this was a good opportunity to try something that would be interesting, that would be fun and educational, and it seemed like it would be a good chance to do something unusual . . . so I took it. And it was all of those things! I was amazingly lucky to have been the first one there and to work with Gertrude Lamb. She was such a special person.

KM: How did the realities of the CML position compare to your initial expectations, going into this new role?
CR: I didn't really have any expectations. I expected things to go well, and they did. I didn't have any idea what the job was going to be like. I showed up for my first day, they showed me an office, and inside I said, "Oh, wow, an office." I hadn't expected that!

KM: So, it seems as if you have a personality that fit very well with this evolving role.
CR: Yes, I've always maintained that flexibility and adaptability are important for searching. . . . The CML activity [requires] a very sophisticated kind of reference [searching], because a lot more is needed from the CML; you have to do a lot more interpreting on your own. Which is good for a reference librarian to do too, interacting with the user, asking questions, and really talking during the reference interview, but some reference librarians don't go

to that extreme. And the fact that we were outside the library, at least half the time, about the only time off and the time we went back to the library was to do the actual searches because at that time searching could only be done on some kind of computer terminal. There wasn't any carrying around your phone, or your iPad, or anything like that. Which is amazing, I can't even imagine what it would be like today! We also spent a lot of time in the outpatient clinic as well as the inpatient floors, and that activity outside the library is what gave us a lot more insight into what was really going on in the daily world of the physicians, the residents, the students, and the other members of the health-care team. We got to know the patients. We recognized, especially in the city hospital, that there were often the same people coming back. As the medical school gained in its reputation, as a quality place to go, there were different kinds of patients as well, but it was still a city hospital. So the type of work that I did was great; it was fascinating, a good opportunity to learn.

KM: Could you tell us a little about your first impressions of Gertrude Lamb, when you first met her?
CR: Honestly, I don't remember when I first met her. I felt like through the years I got to know her so well; I can't separate out my first impression. I can mention the fact that the third day that I was on the job at UMKC, she came to me and she said, "We're all going to a library meeting here in the city, and I think you have been here long enough that you will be able to handle the Circ[ulation] desk by yourself." So, it was those kinds of things, but she was just great to work with. I enjoyed working with her very much. And I enjoyed socializing with her as well. We had our share of parties at UMKC as well, at the library and at various people's houses.

KM: How did Gertrude prepare you, and as they came aboard, other members of the CML team for this new opportunity?
CR: Well she had gone on rounds before I got there, and then she sent me off to go on rounds, and actually relied on me to break in the two new guys. And I actually participated in their interviews, too, for the hiring process, because I was the one who was familiar on a day-to-day basis with what actually went on, on rounds, on the teams, with the students, and so forth. And so I was pretty much responsible for taking care of them and getting them going. And at one point in time I started using the title "senior CML."

KM: And they would come to you with questions before they went to Gertrude?
CR: Yes, if it was about CML stuff. About research activity . . . she [Gertrude Lamb] was the researcher. She did the research, got the grant to start with, initiated our research aspects of the grant. We did a study of the antici-

pated information needs and how well they went. I don't have that study anymore, so I can't discuss the results of that.

KM: Can you talk a bit about the types of questions you received those first few months?
CR: Yes. It wasn't so much that we got questions; it was that we anticipated the information needs. We always got the regular questions such as "what is the best drug to treat this, among these three?" You know, those kinds of things, regular clinical reference questions.

KM: So, as you became more comfortable with the team, and they got to know more about your skills, did you notice any changes to the volume or style of questions asked? Less anticipatory and more direct questions?
CR: Exactly, there was more asking. There was more discussion, and I was more included. . . . There was more camaraderie. As with any team, as they develop and they get to know each other, there is more interaction.

KM: Can you recall any professional opportunities that developed [while a CML] that you did not originally anticipate?
CR: I think that the online searching opportunities that I took advantage of were probably the biggest. The fact that I got to learn it. I got to use it. I got to learn more about it. I got sent off to NLM for classes. I would go to updates, and I got to be recognized as somebody who kind of knew what was going on.

KM: How did Lamb propose to evaluate the impact of the CML program? Obviously as it was grant funded, I'm sure that evaluation was part of the expectations . . .
CR: Yes, for the report. Well . . . hypothesis #1, as I remember, had to do with whether the CMLs could actual identify an unexpressed need. Could they legitimately anticipate needs that were actual needs? How much agreement was there between the CML and the health person, as to the need for information? Another hypothesis was that information systems could be developed, like the LATCH system, like "Current References" or "Current Topics." Could those really be helpful in the patient-care setting? And I honestly don't remember anything about the results except that I understood from my students, especially from my students, that the LATCH system was good. It was also helpful to the nurses. I got feedback, just subjective feedback from the nurses, that they really liked having that information. It wasn't physically attached to the charts; it was in a file in the nurses station, where everyone knew where it was, filed by patient and not subject. So, if you were looking at patient X, you could look up patient X in the file and see articles that had to do with whatever patient X was in there for.

KM: And you pulled those articles and made them available?

CR: Yes: searched, analyzed retrieval, selected articles, made copies, and filed them on the ward.

KM: As the CML service became more established, did you notice any changes in professional respect from your teams, as they became more familiar with your services?

CR: Yes, from "thank you very much but we don't need that service" to "oh, please, please help me!" It was kind of like that.

KM: How did you see the CML role as being understood by other librarians, those who were reference librarians?

CR: Well there was a lot of, well I don't want to say confusion, but a lot of "what's going on?" I can't tell you how many times I explained, how many times I had a little slide show that I would show. We did poster sessions in Minnesota . . . [at MLA's annual meeting in] 1986. We just talked and talked, every year, every time we went to MLA especially, or the chapter meetings, and various places in the mid-continental chapter.

KM: Lamb left UMKC during 1973, to return to Connecticut (where her husband lived and taught). Could you reflect a bit on this transition?

CR: Yes, her husband never moved to Kansas City, so they were having a very long-distance relationship. Her mother lived with her in Kansas City, and her mother was in failing health, and it was a combination of Jack [Lamb's husband] being still in Connecticut and her mother's failing health that made her seek someplace else. Hartford, Storrs is where they were from. And they loved her in Storrs. When I went to her memorial service, and talked to people who had known her in the community, it was great.

KM: That's so nice to hear. And it sounds like, in the two years that she was at UMKC, and in no small part due to you also, she really got the CML program up and running. It seems to have sustained itself because of what you had done.

CR: Well, it was because of what she did. She got it started. She got the grant. She got us going. She hired me; she hired Jim and Russ [UMKC's second and third CMLs]. She got it firmly in place.

KM: And all in two years.

CR: Yes, it really was only about two years.

KM: That is impressive. It really shows her force of will, I think.

CR: Very strong, very strong personality, yes. And she did the same thing in Hartford Hospital. She just kind of went right in and got them going too.

KM: And did you remain in contact with her, after her departure?
CR: Mostly just Christmas cards. We'd see each other at MLA, because that was the place where we would be together. I was hardly ever in Storrs. And even when I moved to the East Coast, I just didn't get up there. But we would see each other at MLA, and have breakfast and get together and talk. She was a great, great person.

In 1973, Gertrude Lamb left UMKC and assumed the role of university assistant librarian and director of Hartford Hospital's clinical librarian program.[27] Despite the loss of their visionary leader, UMKC's CMLs continued. At the MLA annual meeting in 1974, the CML program and its early successes were formally unveiled to the greater medical library community by the new director in the "Report on the Biomedical Librarian in the Patient-Care Setting at the University of Missouri–Kansas City School of Medicine." A component of a larger session on *Information for Patient Care and Medical Education*, the report highlighted impressive results.

Circulation statistics at UMKC rose from a previous high of 1,604 transactions in November 1971 to 3,438 in October 1973.[28] User feedback data reported information selected by the CML addressed specific clinical need 95.3 percent of the time; CML information completely answered questions 65.2 percent of the time with an additional 29.4 percent of information providing nearly complete answers.[29]

University of Connecticut Health Center and Hartford Hospital

Gertrude Lamb established a second clinical program at Connecticut's Hartford Hospital and gained additional NLM funding in support of a research grant titled "Clinical Librarians in the Patient Care Setting."[30] Lamb identified differences between the focus of the UMKC and Hartford CML programs: at UMKC the CMLs focused on education, specifically that of the medical student; at Hartford CMLs provided direct support of patient care with the clinical team for the betterment of the patient.[31] Lamb described Hartford activities as centered around "[professional] acceptance, information delivery, [and] impact on patient care and changes in the information seeking behavior of health care professionals."[32]

Similar to the UMKC experience, an early goal of the Hartford program was establishing professional acceptance of the CML role. Initially viewed as a novelty and chiefly accepted due to clinical team curiosity, CMLs attended bedside rounds, defined clinician information needs, and selected appropriate literature in a timely manner. Successful completion of these tasks furthered the process of acceptance and moved the CML from curiosity to functioning team member.[33] One CML member noted clinicians had explained their routines and defined medical abbreviations at the beginning of her tenure but stopped as trust in her grew. Attending physicians sought CML expertise at times other than during rounds. CMLs joined hospital advisory councils and external medical conferences, further reflecting professional acceptance of the CML.[34]

Identifying professional acceptance of CMLs was achievable, but articulating the impact of other components of Lamb's program proved more difficult. Lamb sought to explore the CML's impact on patient care. Although it was simple (and typical) to quantify the number of literature requests following the addition of a CML to a clinical team, measuring the actual impact of delivered information was much harder. Lamb discussed this conundrum in her oral history and noted at first her team wanted to define and count "impact documents," literature a clinician identified as having either "confirmed or changed patient care."[35] Yet they were unsure how to account for future cases where the same clinician applied to the information. If information benefited development of a hospital treatment protocol, would CMLs count impact on care of future patients affected by the new protocol?

In 1981, Scura and Davidoff created a novel method to appraise impact of CML services. They defined the impact by comparing them to sources of clinical information more familiar to physicians, specifically clinical laboratory tests and X-ray technology.[36] Scura and Davidoff discovered that laboratory tests resulted in treatment-altering data approximately 5 percent of the time, while CML services directly affected patient treatment 20 percent of the time. When looking at impact on diagnostic thinking, CMLs performed favorably when compared to X-ray films, with CML searches resulting in a clinician changing or confirming diagnostic thinking in 86 percent of cases. Additionally, CML services cost much less than a single X-ray or one set of electrolyte studies.[37]

OTHER EARLY CML PROGRAMS AND EVALUATION EFFORTS

Inspired by Lamb's UMKC and Hartford successes, librarians created CML programs at other hospitals and medical schools and reported their impact on clinical knowledge and patient care throughout the 1970s. In 1973, Cedars-Sinai Medical Center in Los Angeles started a small CML service that served the pediatrics and obstetrics departments. Cedars-Sinai CMLs reported how best to identify "good" articles, the need to process daily exposure to illness and death, and the best usage of limited time. Other results included the CML's increased understanding of physician needs and physicians' opinion of the library's ability to address educational goals.[38] In 1974, librarians at the Washington University School of Medicine Library in St. Louis established a CML program where CMLs attended residents' morning report sessions. Residents in that program reported 35 percent of CML search results directly informed patient care.[39] In 1975, the Yale Medical Library expanded their program to provide CML coverage to the departments of pediatrics, psychiatry, internal medicine, and three surgical subspecialties at Yale-New Haven Hospital. Yale CMLs collected questionnaire data that indicated clinicians considered CML search results highly relevant and helpful to patient care.[40]

ROLE NEGOTIATION AND VALIDATION IN A CHANGING HEALTH CARE ENVIRONMENT

The Tax Equity and Fiscal Responsibility Act (PL 97-248) of 1982 charged the Department of Health and Human Services (DHHS) with forming a medical prospective payment system. The legislation created the Health Care Financing Administration (HCFA) that developed a new hospital reimbursement system based on diagnosis-related groups (DRGs) and defined library costs as overhead. In 1983, a Federal Register announcement clarified the HCFA legislation and announced hospitals were no longer required to maintain libraries in order to receive reimbursement for Medicare/Medicaid patients.[41] HCFA's Final Rule in 1984 prohibited classifying medical library costs as part of the hospital's medical education's costs.[42]

In 1990, the Joint Commission introduced its "Agenda for Change" and in 1994 published its first accreditation manual that eliminated departmental requirements and moved to organizational functions.[43] The 1994 Joint Commission standards organized library functions under the broad umbrella of information management (IM).[44] The Joint Commission identified four different types of data covered by the IM standard, including literature or "knowledge-based information." IM standard 9 (IM.9) described parameters for use of knowledge-based information and asserted, "An organization is not required to have a library." This, along with the omission of *librarians* from the Joint Commission's professional grid and lack of definition of "professional hospital librarian" in the *Interpretation of Terms* glossary,[45] could have led hospital administrators to believe librarians and libraries were no longer necessary.

MLA responded to these changes in accreditation standards by forming a Joint Commission Information Management Task Force (Task Force). Charged with advising the Joint Commission on ramifications of the revisited standards, Task Force members addressed opportunities created for medical librarians specifically emphasizing the value CMLs provided clinical teams.[46] Schardt amplified the Task Force message by outlining opportunities for medical librarians in nearly every chapter of the revised Joint Commission standards.[47]

Today Joint Commission standards follow the same organizational function format, and demonstrating the value CMLs deliver to health-care teams and patients remains important. CMLs provide many services including providing patient and family education, improving organizational performance with tools for leadership, management of human resources, management of the environment of care, surveillance, and prevention and control of infection, in addition to the critical role of managing information and delivering timely knowledge based information in support of patient care.

PATIENT CARE OUTCOMES REVISITED

HCFA's Final Rule renewed CML's efforts to quantify their value through a series of research studies. Two seminal studies broke ground with significant documentation of hospital libraries' contributions to patient care. David King evaluated the impact of librarian-provided information on clinicians.[48] Using King's methodology, the Rochester study focused on physicians' perceptions of library information on decision-making.[49] Other studies and systematic reviews conducted between 1992 and 2011 sought to measure the value and types of information provided by libraries.[50] Two studies provided evidence that hospital length of stay decreased at hospitals with medical library service.[51] Jemison et al. developed a return on investment (ROI) tool for the Department of Veterans Affairs (VA) libraries.[52] Dunn et al. laid groundwork to update and repeat the Rochester study with a larger number of participating facilities, and Marshall et al. reported on the results of this study.[53] Jones et al. conducted a study of VA libraries between 2006 and 2008 that adopted several concepts from the Rochester study to identify ROI for VA library programs.[54]

BACK TO THE BEDSIDE: REFINED ROLES, NOVEL TITLES

In 1985, Covell questioned *if* clinicians in professional practice received appropriate and reliable information.[55] Later that year Gorman examined *how* clinicians used information.[56] Subsequent studies delved into the types of questions asked when clinicians see patients.[57] These studies revealed that each patient visit generates one to two clinical questions. Academic medical centers and teaching hospitals create a higher volume of clinical questions, an average of five per patient, and encourage development of CML programs. The outcome of these studies validated benefits of the CML and helped pave the way for more automated information delivery mechanisms in patient records.[58]

Convinced of the need for bedside information professionals, Nunzia Giuse, a physician and librarian, at the Eskind Biomedical Library (EBL) of Vanderbilt University Medical Center established an ambitious CML program in 1996. Vanderbilt's CML program represented a major realignment in library services. All librarians working at EBL, including those involved with circulation and technical services, participated in clinical rounds.[59] During the transition period, CMLs chose specific clinical specialties they preferred to support. EBL administrators evaluated searching skills of librarians and provided financial support for additional training and continuing educational activities. CMLs learned methods of critical appraisal and skills to write concise synopses of medical literature and earned an equal voice on clinical teams.[60] Through intense professional mentorship, clinical education, and administrative championing, Giuse promoted a vision of a clinical information professional and developed a formal entrance to the bedside for CMLs. In many ways, this foreshadowed the informationist model proposed by clinical researchers Davidoff and Florance.

The Informationist Rises

Studies consistently identified the clinician's reliance on medical information for evidence-based, point-of-care information. In 1997, Davidoff and Florance published an editorial that described a new health professional called the "informationist" and identified questions that "can, and should, be answered on the basis of evidence from the published literature" but remain unaddressed because physicians do not have the time or skills to seek out answers themselves.[61] Davidoff and Florance's informationist provides answers to clinical questions in real time; the authors proposed establishment of a "national program, modeled on the experience of clinical librarianship, to train, credential, and pay for the services of information specialists."[62] Informationists would be trained in information science and "domain knowledge," an area of clinical expertise. Expectations of the informationist role include a core knowledge base of basic medical concepts, principles of clinical epidemiology, biostatistics, critical appraisal, and information management. Davidoff and Florance championed the Vanderbilt model as a supervised practicum for informationists and suggested training programs be accredited and graduates certified through a national agency.[63]

Reaction from the library community was mixed. Some argued creators of the informationist concept did not fully explore or appreciate the ability and value of CMLs.[64] Other stakeholders, like the National Institutes of Health (NIH) Library welcomed the new role and developing a national program that embedded informationists at sixteen labs or clinics in Health and Human Services agency offices. Significant events in the history of the informationist program include a national conference[65] and formal definition of the role and publication of a case study.[66] The informationist concept and popularity increased in well-funded academic institutions that were able to offer such a specialty program.

AND ONWARD, THE CML AND INFORMATIONIST OF TODAY

Davidoff and Florance challenged the medical profession to embrace the informationist role as a way to link biomedical medical literature to the patient at the point of care. A quarter century earlier, Gertrude Lamb and her associates encouraged clinicians to accept clinical medical librarians for much the same reason. Despite the forceful advocacy of these towering figures, decades of research reporting positively on information impact, and thousands of current CML/informationist professionals active in medical centers, the CML role remains underutilized and undervalued. There is no standard CML or informationist presence in hospitals across the United States even though missing literature can cause costly mistakes or, as in the case of a clinical trial at Johns Hopkins in 2001, even death.[67]

Since Lamb's time, well-connected library leaders who understand the vital nature of these roles and are passionate about the information professional's role in patient care work to keep them relevant by responding to organizational needs. Visionary leaders flexibly adapt CML programs as standards change and, more importantly, as health-care priorities and needs for information change. Developing opportunities for CMLs include: gaining access to the electronic medical record, providing specialized information services to enable hospitals to achieve Magnet status, responding to the changing nature of evidence-based medicine in medical education, selecting and creatively introducing digital content and tools to provide clinicians with point-of-care information, expanding consumer health services, and participating in public health initiatives.

While variability among programs contributed to difficulties measuring impact, history shows that local adaptability is a positive and a defining trait of clinical medical librarianship. By weaving opportunities into their daily practice, information professionals continue to adapt. The provision of point-of-care information is individualistic by nature and bound to the unique needs of our patrons. Historically CMLs relied on specific knowledge of patron needs to improve and enhance patient care and clinical decision-making, and chances are CMLs will continue to do so.

NOTES

1. Gertrude Lamb, interview by Estelle Brodman, Medical Library Association Oral History Committee (1985).
2. Lamb, interview.

3. L. A. Colaianni, "Hospital Librarians and the Medical Library Association," *Bull Med Libr Assoc* 86, no. 2 (1998).

4. L. Darling, "Changes in Information Delivery since 1960 in Health Sciences Libraries," *Library Trends* (1974).

5. L. S. Sutton and P. A. Wolfgram, "Hospital Libraries in the United States: Historical Antecedents," *Bull Med Libr Assoc* 73, no. 1 (1985).

6. A. Bunting, "The Nation's Health Information Network: History of the Regional Medical Library Program, 1965–1985," *Bull Med Libr Assoc* 75, no. 3 Suppl (1987).

7. S. L. Speaker, "An Historical Overview of the National Network of Libraries of Medicine, 1985–2015," *J Med Libr Assoc* 106, no. 2 (2018).

8. Sutton and Wolfgram, "Hospital Libraries in the United States."

9. M. Young, "Latch Brings Medical Literature to Patient's Bedside," *Crossreference* 5, no. 8 (1975).

10. S. L. Sowell, "Latch at the Washington Hospital Center, 1967–1975," *Bull Med Libr Assoc* 66, no. 2 (1978).

11. Sowell, "Latch at the Washington Hospital Center."

12. S. A. Hargrave, "Latch—It Works!" *Hosp Libr* 1, no. 5 (1976); L. A. Brenner, "Report on LATCH (Literature Attached to Charts)," *Med Rec News* 47, no. 30 (1976).

13. C. C. Nippert, "Online Latch," *Med Ref Serv Q* 4, no. 1 (1985).

14. E. G. Detlefsen, "Gertrude H. Lamb, 1918-2015, AHIP, FMLA," *J Med Libr Assoc* 103, no. 2 (2015).

15. Lamb, interview.

16. V. Algermissen, "Biomedical Librarians in a Patient Care Setting at the University of Missouri-Kansas City School of Medicine," *Bull Med Libr Assoc* 62, no. 4 (1974).

17. Algermissen, "Biomedical Librarians in a Patient Care Setting ."

18. Lamb, interview.

19. Lamb, interview.

20. Lamb, interview.

21. Algermissen, "Biomedical Librarians in a Patient Care Setting."

22. Algermissen, "Biomedical Librarians in a Patient Care Setting."

23. Algermissen, "Biomedical Librarians in a Patient Care Setting."

24. Lamb, interview.

25. Lamb, interview.

26. Lamb, interview.

27. Detlefsen, "Gertrude H. Lamb."

28. Algermissen, "Biomedical Librarians in a Patient Care Setting."

29. G. G. Claman, "Clinical Medical Librarians: What They Do and Why," *Bull Med Libr Assoc* 73, no. 1 (Jan 1985).

30. Detlefsen, "Gertrude H. Lamb."

31. Lamb, interview.

32. G. Lamb, "Bridging the Information Gap," *Hosp Libr* 1, no. 10 (1976).

33. G. Lamb, "Bridging the Information Gap."

34. G. Lamb, "Bridging the Information Gap."

35. G. Lamb, "Bridging the Information Gap."

36. G. Scura and F. Davidoff, "Case-Related Use of the Medical Literature. Clinical Librarian Services for Improving Patient Care," *JAMA* 245, no. 1 (1985).

37. Scura and Davidoff, "Case-Related Use of the Medical Literature."

38. L. A. Colaianni, "Clinical Medical Librarians in a Private Teaching-Hospital Setting," *Bull Med Libr Assoc* 63, no. 4 (1975).

39. C. B. Staudt, B. Halbrook, and E. Brodman, "A Clinical Librarians' Program—an Attempt at Evaluation," *Bull Med Libr Assoc* 64, no. 2 (1976).

40. B. Greenberg, S. Barrison, M. Kolisch, and M, Leredu, "Evaluation of a Clinical Medical Librarian Program at the Yale Medical Library," *Bull Med Libr Assoc* 66, no. 3 (1978).

41. *Tax Equity and Fiscal Responsibility Act,* Public Law 97-248, *U.S. Statutes at Large* 96.324 (1982).

42. "Proposed Rules: Medical Library," *Fed Reg* 48(2), 42CFR19:305.

43. V. J. McLarney, "'Agenda for Change' Focuses on Quality Assurance," *Health Facil Manage*, 2, no. 7 (1989); D. Fogg, "Discussion of the Joint Commission on Accreditation of Healthcare Organizations' Agenda for Change," *AORN J* 58 no. 2 (1993).

44. J. D. Doyle, "Knowledge-Based Information Management: Implications for Information Services," *Med Ref Serv Q* 13, no. 2 (1994).

45. P. W. Dalrymple and C. S. Scherrer, "Tools for Improvement: A Systematic Analysis and Guide to Accreditation by the JCAHO," *Bull Med Libr Assoc* 86, no. 1 (1998).

46. Doyle, "Knowledge-Based Information Management"; J. Bradley, "Management of Information: Analysis of the Joint Commission's Standards for Information Management," *Top Health Inf Manage* 16, no. 2 (1995); C. J. Jones, "Charting a Path for Health Sciences Librarians in an Integrated Information Environment," *Bull Med Libr Assoc* 81, no. 4 (1993).

47. C. M. Schardt, "Going Beyond Information Management: Using the Comprehensive Accreditation Manual for Hospitals to Promote Knowledge-Based Information Services," *Bull Med Libr Assoc* 86 (1998).

48. D. N. King, "The Contribution of Hospital Library Information Services to Clinical Care: A Study in Eight Hospitals," *Bull Med Libr Assoc* 75 (1987).

49. J. G. Marshall, "The Impact of the Hospital Library on Clinical Decision Making: The Rochester Study," *Bull Med Libr Assoc* 80, no. 2 (1992); "Measuring the Value and Impact of Health Library and Information Services: Past Reflections, Future Possibilities," *Health Info Libr J* 24 Suppl 1 (2007).

50. W. W. Fischer and L. B. Reel, "Total Quality Management (TQM) in a Hospital Library: Identifying Service Benchmarks," *Bull Med Libr Assoc* 80, no. 4 (1992); A. Brettle et al., "Evaluating Clinical Librarian Services: A Systematic Review," *Health Info Libr J* 28, no. 1 (2011).

51. M. A. Banks, "Defining the Informationist: A Case Study from the Frederick L. Ehrman Medical Library," *J Med Libr Assoc* 94, no. 1 (2006); M. S. Klein, F. V. Ross, D. L. Adams, and C. M. Gilbert, "Effect of Online Literature Searching on Length of Stay and Patient Care Costs," *Acad Med* 69, no. 6 (1994).

52. K. Jemison et al., "Measuring Return on Investment in VA Libraries," *J Hosp Libr* 9, no. 4 (2009).

53. K. Dunn et al., "Measuring the Value and Impact of Health Sciences Libraries: Planning an Update and Replication of the Rochester Study," *J Med Libr Assoc* 97, no. 4 (2009); J. G. Marshall et al., "The Value of Library and Information Services in Patient Care: Results of a Multisite Study," *J Med Libr Assoc* 101, no. 1 (2013).

54. D. A. Jones, E. J. Poletti, and P. Stephenson, "Demonstrating the Value of Library Services in South Center VA Health Care Network Medical Centers," *J Hosp Librsh* 10, no. 3 (2010).

55. D. G. Covell, G. C. Uman, and P. R. Manning, "Information Needs in Office Practice: Are They Being Met?" *Ann Intern Med* no. 4 (1985).

56. P. N. Gorman, J. Ash, and L. Wykoff, "Can Primary Care Physicians' Questions Be Answered Using the Medical Journal Literature?" *Bull Med Libr Assoc* 82, no. 2 (1994).

57. G. Del Fiol, T. E. Workman, and P. N. Gorman, "Clinical Questions Raised by Clinicians at the Point of Care: A Stystematic Review," *JAMA Intern Med* 174, no. 5 (2014).

58. J. A. Osheroff et al., "Physicians' Information Needs: Analysis of Questions Posed During Clinical Teaching," *Ann Intern Med* 114, no. 7 (1991); D. E. Forsythe, B. G. Buchanan, J. A. Osheroff, and R. A. Miller, "Expanding the Concept of Medical Information: An Observational Study of Physicians' Information Needs," *Comput Biomed Res* 25, no. 2 (1992).

59. N. B. Giuse, "Advancing the Practice of Clinical Medical Librarianship," *Bull Med Libr Assoc* 85, no. 4 (1997).

60. Giuse, "Advancing the Practice of Clinical Medical Librarianship."

61. F. Davidoff and V. Florance, "The Informationist: A New Health Profession?" *Bull Med Libr Assoc* 85, no. 4 (1997).

62. Davidoff and Florance, "The Informationist."

63. Giuse, "Advancing the Practice of Clinical Medical Librarianship"; N. B. Giuse et al., "Advancing the Practice of Clinical Medical Librarianship," *Bull Med Libr Assoc* 85 no. 4 (1997).

64. D. G. Wolf et al., "Hospital Librarianship in the United States: At the Crossroad," *J Med Libr Assoc* 90, no. 1 (2002).

65. J. P. Shipman, D. J. Cunningham, R. Holst, and L. A. Watson, "The Informationist Conference: Report," *J Med Libr Assoc*, no. 4.

66. M. A. Banks, "Defining the Informationist: A Case Study from the Frederick L. Ehrman Medical Library," *J Med Libr Assoc* 94, no. 1 (2006); K. B. Oliver and N. K. Roderer, "Working Towards the Informationist," *Health Informatics J* 12, no. 1 (2006).

67. S. Ramsay, "Johns Hopkins Takes Responsibility for Volunteer's Death," *Lancet* 358, no. 9277 (2001); R. Steinbrook, "Protecting Research Subjects—the Crisis at Johns Hopkins," *N Engl J Med* 346, no. 9 (2002).

Chapter Two

Creating Clinical Partnerships

Judy C. Stribling and Antonio P. DeRosa

GETTING STARTED

If you are a newly minted librarian, a fresh hire to an institution, or even an old pro charged with expanding an existing medical library program, establishing partnerships and creating good rapport with clinicians, clinical departments, professors, and high-level administrators is imperative for success. Librarians can expect to achieve great results and high levels of support if they understand the importance of creating value-added services for clinicians that improve patient safety and quality of care and ultimately result in increased patient satisfaction. Successful "boundary spanning," the ability to reach across borders, build relationships, and manage complex issues and information, is a core activity for health science librarians. Humphreys eloquently describes the need for librarians to "bridge internal silos and reach across borders within the larger institutions that they serve as well as with outside groups, disciplines, and organizations."[1]

Silos exist to protect the status quo. Your mission is to introduce new advancements in services to existing customers and build new customer bases, not maintain the status quo. How do you become an effective change agent in environments resistant to transformation? Creating transformational partnerships requires strategic planning. In order to build and move forward, you must first understand your customers and identify how you are meeting or failing to meet their needs. Do this by *actively listening* to your customers and aligning your program with the end goal of meeting and exceeding their requirements.

IDENTIFY MAJOR PLAYERS AND STAKEHOLDERS

Medical librarians, usually referred to as clinical medical librarians (CMLs), work in a variety of institutions at different levels, with different job descriptions and for different populations. In general, the CML's role is to provide information to clinicians, other health-care providers, and patients, and to assist in improving clinician's information-seeking skills.[2] The most common work environments for CMLs are hospitals, medical schools, nursing schools, and academic medical centers (AMCs). Each of these institutions has unique needs, missions, and key clinical stakeholders. AMCs comprise all, or most, of the key clinical stakeholders of the other institutions and are the institutional model used in this chapter to guide CMLs to build solid customer bases and relationships.

Most AMCs include a medical school and a hospital where medical college faculty and residents, interns, and fellows practice medicine and medical students complete clinical workshops. The medical school's leader is typically a dean. The hospital leader is usually a dean as well, but not always, and carries the title of president or chief executive officer (CEO). Many medical school faculty have dual appointments to both the college and the hospital. Medical school faculty who lead some departments within the hospital generally have professorial and hospital titles such as "Full Professor of the Medical School and Director of Clinical Department." Residents and interns conduct rounds with attendings and report to full-time faculty. Medical students rotate through different departments throughout their educational curriculum. Other hospital departments report directly to the president, CEO, or middle management under those lines. Nursing programs are almost always managed under hospital leadership. Nurses may report to a vice president of nursing through channels of charge nurses or patient-care directors (PCDs). Identifying the roles of executives, managers, patient coordinators, and so on, and making sure you appreciate the organizational structure is necessary to understand your customer base.

Executives such as deans or CEOs define the culture of an organization and influence value and mission statements. Pay careful attention to the words used by leadership and the leadership's strategic plan. Align your program with the dean's strategy for the school and the educational curriculum for the students. Echoing the message from the top by adjusting or adapting services creates possibilities for dynamic partnerships. Academically, a CML can explore opportunities to teach in the educational curriculum, conduct research, and assist other faculty with research, as well as attend journal clubs and publish with faculty, students, residents, interns, and nurses. The interests and goals of a hospital president or CEO might differ from those of a dean, so a good CML must tweak search strategies and develop plans to satisfy a customer base with varied administrative and multiple management concerns.

CMLs involved in the academic programs of medical and nursing schools teach evidence-based medicine (EBM) in the classroom and support evidence-based practice (EBP) on clinical floors, assist faculty, residents, nurses, and students with publishing efforts, and conduct systematic reviews. Identify the individuals in charge of EBM and EBP for departments. Similarly, CMLs work in clinical operations in academic medical centers, hospitals, medical schools, and nursing schools where physicians/faculty, hospitalists, chief residents, charge nurses, or PCDs usually lead the day-to-day clinical operations on hospital floors accompanied by CMLs. While participating in clinical operations with a team, observe the individuals. Who is the most or least welcoming member of the team to you? Either one of them may become your greatest fan. Pay attention to the personalities of everyone around you. Get to know who has a good sense of humor, who is the group grump, who asks the most questions. You never know who might become your future partner or champion.

Conduct a thorough review of which library services and programs are available to a customer before meeting with him or her. You want to enter meetings already knowing about past problems, complaints, or instances when the library's performance was viewed as less than stellar. You can manage problems by correcting services, amending service requirements, abandoning services altogether, or suggesting more realistic new service initiatives. Assessing clinical services is an ongoing effort discussed in depth later in this chapter. For now, let us summarize by saying you should conduct a quick under-the-hood look at current services. Arm yourself with a tight elevator pitch[3] that clearly outlines your and your program's unique attributes, skills, and abilities. Get used to revising those pitches as you continue to meet new colleagues and anticipate additional challenges and projects.

When visiting a happy client, ask what is going right. Which services do they value most? What new service would they like to see? Perhaps you demonstrated the collaborative features of a pdf manager to one of the residents during rounds and she liked it. Your next step may be to schedule a demonstration of the technology to the entire department. Do not make a rookie mistake of promising services you are unable to deliver, and make sure you are meeting all realistic requirements. If you are not attending the department's Grand Rounds, put it on your calendar and go. Does the department have morning report? At what time does it occur, and does it fit into your or your team's schedule? If so, ask for permission to attend.

Build strong relationships with the administrative staff of your customers. Administrative assistants are gatekeepers and valuable information banks. They control calendars, schedule appointments, and usually know most of the moving parts of the organization. When faced with a crucial need for assistance or information, having a strong working relationship with administrative staff can be a deal maker or breaker. Imagine you are scheduled to present a new product to the department chair and faculty. The meeting is taking place in a seldom-used conference room. You have the room number and feel confident you can find it, but in fact, you cannot. The path to the room is a maze, and there are no breadcrumbs to help you find your way. A quick call to an assistant, who answers your call because he knows you, solves your problem. You make it to the hidden lair on time and enjoy adding another building geography victory to your belt! Networking with administrative assistants can help you with challenges other than giving directions or getting valuable time on someone's calendar. Having an ally in an administrative role may gain you access to highly visible institutional events and provide opportunities to rub elbows with clients in different environments.

Stepping Out

Attend every open event your schedule allows. Lectures, grand rounds, or other functions where clinicians gather are great places to introduce yourself and the services you offer. This part of relationship-building is seeing and being seen.

Vignette

Recently, co-author DeRosa attended an annual hospital kick-off meeting. The hospital's CEO and COO presented their plans and goals for the next year to an audience of almost three thousand people. At the end of the presentation, they took turns answering audience questions. Seeing an opportunity to raise awareness of librarian expertise in clinical care, DeRosa asked a thoughtful question about patient health literacy in underserved populations in some of the satellite neighborhoods of Brooklyn and Queens that the academic medical center serves. Seeing himself on the big screen in a large midtown ballroom, DeRosa joked that he appreciates the screen time opportunity. This led to laugher by the attendees and both the CEO and COO. The CEO responded in a joking way about the width of DeRosa's tie. DeRosa parlayed the tie comment in such a way that made it clear the CEO, not the COO, had to answer his question. Throughout the Q&A, the CEO and COO bantered back and forth about who would answer each question. This simple action on the part of DeRosa had great impact. Since that event, several researchers have approached DeRosa, and one wrote him into a grant dealing with a decision navigation intervention to assist newly diagnosed prostate cancer patients in Brooklyn and Queens communities.

DeRosa's experience illustrates the value in showing up and demonstrating your professional credentials. This is an exciting time for CMLs. We increasingly play pivotal roles in clinical research, patient-centered care, and community outreach and patient-engagement research projects.[4] CMLs do more than understand researchers' needs for standard library services of information search and retrieval. We suggest innovative technology services to manage information, anticipate new demands for data management and storage, and work collaboratively with colleagues in information technology (IT) and bio-informatics. We also help researchers meet growing challenges of sharing, managing, and preserving ever-growing amounts of data.[5]

DEVELOP AN ONLINE PRESENCE

Make sure your electronic presence reflects the image you wish to convey to existing and future clients. Developing a polished and consistent web presence is no easy task, but it is worth spending the time and effort to finesse. As current medical students, faculty, and clinicians are entering the health-care field, you can bet that most of them are super users when it comes to the internet. After all, many of these practitioners are of the generation who grew up with the internet.[6] These digital immigrants and natives require a customized approach to delivery of information. If clinical medical librarians cannot rise to the challenge and meet the needs of these tech-savvy users, it will be difficult to relate to them and "sell" the myriad services and resources that can benefit their clinical practice.

CMLs should be focusing efforts on developing seamless access to point-of-care tools and other evidence-based medicine resources. This should transcend the usual computer terminal/desktop approach to accessing information, and encompass directions on accessing tools from mobile and hand-held devices.[7] LibGuides and library websites seem to be the standard platform for curating mobile resources related to clinical practice. It is important to be as descriptive as possible in the instructions for accessing these resources. CMLs should also remember that in the changing digital landscape, permalinks and instructions for mobile resource access change rapidly. Setting up a schedule to update LibGuides and websites on a regular basis will help to alleviate some of the stressors that go into keeping current with key access points for major databases and resources.[8]

In addition to offering accessible information to clinical partners, having an intuitive web presence of all clinical information services available to clinicians is another must. Providing clinical users with a "one-stop shop," not only for accessing key resources but also for learning more about what the CML can do for them and how CML's expertise can be leveraged to enhance their clinical work, is a good idea. Since the 1990s, library websites have evolved from the simple pathfinder model to the more robust and user-centric portal for all of a user's information needs.[9] Since a library website can be viewed as a marketing tool with customized user experiences built in, it is no surprise that more and more health sciences libraries are developing user-specific webpages containing information of particular interest to given groups or departments. CMLs should be taking advantage of the past decade's renaissance of the library website and developing content that caters to the unique needs of their clinical partners. Included in this is the addition of social media platforms to highlight clinical projects and research and elevate the engagement of clinical information services.[10] Developing a task force or committee within your health sciences library to evaluate the needs and potential impact of a social media presence as an addition to your already-established web presence of clinical information services is a good first step.

LEVERAGE EVIDENCE-BASED MEDICINE

Librarians do not passively wait in the stacks for health-care providers to ask for assistance with clinical questions. Gertrude Lamb's pioneers made a gigantic leap forward to place CMLs on hospital floors in interactive roles with clinicians. CMLs were integrated further into the clinical realm as practitioners gradually accepted EBM as a standard of medical practice. Coined by researchers at McMaster's University in the early 1990s, EBM is "a systemic approach to analyze published research as the basis of clinical decision making." EBM was further refined in 1996 as "the conscientious and judicious use of current best evidence from clinical care research in the management of individual patients."[11] CMLs were early adopters and advocates of the practice, helping it become the international standard. EBM is now a component of most medical schools' curricula, and literature overwhelmingly demonstrates CMLs support EBM training in a variety of capacities.[12] Most models pair a CML with clinical faculty to design EBM courses. This is a prime opportunity to build a strong relationship with a clinician. Demonstrate your skills and promote all EBM products and resources provided by the library.

Teaching medical students provides the opportunity for creating relationships that can last for many years. Open your door to medical students. No matter how smart they think they are, you know things they do not! Being approachable and willing to help them will pay off when students know they can turn to you for assistance. Look for teachable moments during clinical rounds, drawing on these bedside moments as lessons later in the classroom.

Supporting Clinical Research

Perhaps the most apparent and one of the most pivotal services that CMLs should offer clinical partners is stellar clinical searching and literature search support. In this section, the authors walk through a use case for offering literature and clinical question searching support to clinicians. A starting point for delivering this level of service is a simple worksheet that details the process of conducting a thorough search of the literature on a given topic. (See figure 2.1.) A custom search strategy worksheet such as this not only is a good tool for educating clinicians on searching best practices but also provides helpful talking points to assist in the standard reference interview. Of course, in the clinical setting, the reference interview is often abbreviated, so it is even more important to know the relevant questions to ask when you have limited time with a busy clinician. Using a worksheet (or other document) as a guide will help your own clinical practice, and will be appreciated by your clinical team, as it demonstrates your preparedness and respect for your clinical team's time.

You might find that your clinicians are very receptive to learning about the syntax that goes into searching the literature. By opening their eyes to the multitude of advanced ways to search databases, you shed light on other possible partnerships between you and your clinical partners. A search strategy worksheet can contain a step-by-step process for searching and images for easy learning like the one we have developed at Weill Cornell Medicine, or it may follow a different scheme. Although our worksheet serves as a primer for more nuanced clinical searching techniques, the search strategy worksheet presented here is more appropriate for general-purpose questions. The best practice for searching clinical questions is the PICO.[13] The PICO framework is an acronym for: Patient(s)/Population(s), Intervention(s), Comparator(s), Outcome(s). It is a guideline for helping learners understand the major concepts in clinical questions or patient-care scenarios.

To support the clinical scenario and patient-care information needs of clinicians, CMLs may consider the use of more clinically focused databases and decision-support tools. For instance, PubMed's "Clinical Queries" section offers robust searching capabilities on a number of clinical topics.[14] "Clinical Queries" strives to provide comprehensive information and the highest levels of evidence in clinical research areas. Through validated search filters and hedges, "Clinical Queries" retrieves clinical study publication types and other evidence-based research in the published literature such as systematic reviews and meta-analyses. CMLs should educate and direct clinical users to a resource like "Clinical Queries" to ensure that they are incorporating evidence-based medicine techniques into their everyday practice. Having the knowledge and skills to use a clinical searching resource like "Clinical Queries" to answer patient-care questions will serve clinical partners well today and in the future, whether they end up at a bustling academic medical center or a rural primary care practice and regardless of institutional budgets or fiscal landscapes.

REMAIN CURRENT

To stay informed of developments in the field, CMLs regularly attend national professional conferences, network with colleagues, initiate self-learning, and complete CML courses. We are on the lookout for new information technologies and information management systems to increase efficiencies. We are change agents, and our duty is to share advances with clinicians and medical students. Consider the changes 3D printing brought to medicine and the role librarians played in introducing this technology to clinicians and students. Although it seems so current, 3D printing technology is actually over thirty years old. As the cost of 3D technology fell, medical libraries offered access to the printers to students and academicians. Wagner describes a near perfect instance where an interdisciplinary partnership of biomedical engineers, occupational therapists, and medical librarians introduced a 3D printer to a campus for creation of assistive devices for patients.[15] Now 3D printing is widely incorporated into academic curricula, residency training, and much of health care.

ASSESS PROGRAM

Accrediting and licensing entities require all medical schools and some hospitals to maintain libraries. It is not enough to be required. To thrive, libraries and librarians must demonstrate value and illustrate positive impact on institutional missions to gain stakeholders' enthusiastic substantive support. Good practice requires occasional informal checks and balances of services and programs. Planning longitudinal assessments of services and programs is more likely to deliver quality results in the end.[16] Library literature is rich with descriptions of assessment plans used by librarians to measure and benchmark programs. CML program assessments show that CMLs on clinical rounds add to the culture of learning, assist in formation of good clinical questions, and improve student search strategies,[17] and that personal contact with CMLs increases confidence in the search results delivered.[18] Notably, a 2013 landmark study revealed library and information resources had an impact on patient care.[19]

Proving success requires metrics. Measuring numbers of questions answered, information delivered, and time and resources used is relatively easy to do. But you must record the same deliverable every day, year after year to demonstrate effect. Create additional data points as needed. Through numbers and data points, many stories emerge, but subjective storylines may need a different, more anecdotal form of assessment. Delve into qualitative research, and find established survey tools you can easily adapt for your institution and population, or build your own. Face-to-face check-in with

Weill Cornell Medicine
Samuel J. Wood Library

Search Strategy Worksheet

STEP 1: WRITE DOWN RESEARCH TOPIC

Write out your topic in sentence form. For example, *what are the adverse effects of dopamine for treating depressed youth?*

_____

_____

_____

STEP 2: IDENTIFY THE MAJOR CONCEPTS AND DEVELOP LIST OF SEARCH TERMS

Identify and separate your concepts using the headers in the table below. Use the space below the headers to write out any synonyms or alternate terms for the major concepts. Connect terms using the operators (**AND**, **OR**) provided to build your search statement (*see Step 3B for syntax help*). **Hint:** A thesaurus may help when thinking of synonymous terms for your concepts.

	AND		AND		AND	
OR _____		OR _____		OR _____		OR _____
OR _____		OR _____		OR _____		OR _____
OR _____		OR _____		OR _____		OR _____
OR _____		OR _____		OR _____		OR _____
OR _____		OR _____		OR _____		OR _____
OR _____		OR _____		OR _____		OR _____

STEP 3: KNOW YOUR LIMITS (A) AND SYNTAX (B)

(A) Before beginning your search in a database with your specified terms, you should first identify what limits you would like your results to be within. Use the table below as a guide for specifying searching limits. **Note:** limits differ depending on the database; some may have all the limits listed below while others may have fewer.

LIMITS	OPTIONS
Age Limitations	O No Restriction O Newborn (0-1 mo) O Infant (2-23 mos) O Preschool (2 -5 yrs) O Child (6 - 12 yrs) O Adolescent (13 – 18 yrs) O Adult (19 – 44 yrs) O Middle Age (45 – 64 yrs) O Aged (65 + yrs)
Gender	O Male × Female O No Limitations
Species	O Human × Animal O No Limitations
Time Frame	O Current Year O Current Year +5 O Current Year +10 O No Limitations
Languages	O English only O No Limitations O Specific Language _____
Publications	O Comprehensive Search (no limitations) O Review Articles only O Other Publication Specifications _____

Updated: Jan. 2018

Figure 2.1.   Search Strategy Worksheet

(B) Inputting your search terms into a search box properly is crucial to conduct an effective search. See the chart below for a visual of how the Boolean Operators work within most databases.

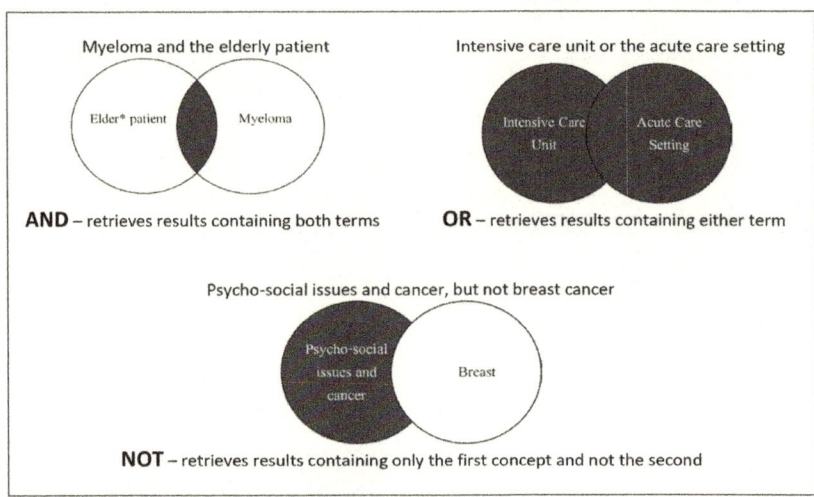

STEP 4: DEVELOP QUERY AND SEARCH THE DATABASE

Use the operators above to develop a logical search query using the terms you specified in step #2.

_____

_____

_____

_____

_____

_____

Updated: Jan. 2018

Figure 2.2.   Search Strategy Worksheet (cont'd)

clients never goes out of style and is key to maintaining strong relationships. Schedule regular meetings with clients if you can. Some clients are just too busy, and it is best to get a sense of how things are going from them during informal elevator bump-ins, collegial chatter before grand rounds, or morning report. Make appropriate adaptations to your services based on feedback from your customers, and continue to enjoy strong relationships.

Creating productive CML team services requires planning and maintaining momentum, and accepting positive results may take time. Successful CML program characteristics are based on mutual respect, clearly defined expectations, innovative practices, consistent communication, and adaptive assessments.

NOTES

1. B. L. Humphreys, "How to Earn a Reputation as a Great Partner," *J Med Libr Assoc* 106, no. 4 (2018).

2. C. E. Lipscomb, "Clinical Librarianship," *Bull Med Libr Assoc* 88, no. 4 (2000); Judy C. Stribling, Keith C. Mages, and Diana Delgado, "Patient-Centered Rounding in an Inpatient Pediatric Setting," *Journal of Hospital Librarianship* 17, no. 2 (2017).

3. Debra Kachel, "Using Research in Talking Points and Elevator Speeches," *Teacher Librarian* 43, no. 1 (2015).

4. Hannah Spring, "Innovation, Engagement and Development: Moving Forward in Health Information Settings," *Health Information & Libraries Journal* (2018).

5. Amalia Monroe-Gulick, Greta Valentine, and Jamene Brooks-Kieffer, "'You Need to Have a Street Beat': A Qualitative Study of Faculty Research Needs and Challenges," *portal: Libraries and the Academy* 17, no. 4 (2017); Kevin B. Read, "Adapting Data Management Education to Support Clinical Research Projects in an Academic Medical Center," *Journal of the Medical Library Association: JMLA* 107, no. 1 (2019).

6. Jeff Urban, "How Growing Up with the Internet Made Millennials Different," *Entrepreneur* (2015), www.entrepreneur.com/article/247886.

7. Jill T. Boruff and Dale Storie, "Mobile Devices in Medicine: A Survey of How Medical Students, Residents, and Faculty Use Smartphones and Other Mobile Devices to Find Information," *Journal of the Medical Library Association: JMLA* 102, no. 1 (2014).

8. Theresa Westbrock, "Reaching Out with Libguides: Establishing a Working Set of Best Practices Au—Gonzalez, Alisa C," *Journal of Library Administration* 50, nos. 5–6 (2010).

9. Stewart M. Brower, "Academic Health Sciences Library Website Navigation: An Analysis of Forty-One Websites and Their Navigation Tools," *Journal of the Medical Library Association: JMLA* 92, no. 4 (2004); Fatemeh Nooshinfard and Soraya Ziaei, "Academic Library Websites as Marketing Tools," *Library Philosophy and Practice*, no. 5-2011 (2011), https://digitalcommons.unl.edu/cgi/viewcontent.cgi?article=1631&context=libphilprac; Karen R. Diaz, "The Role of the Library Web Site: A Step Beyond Deli Sandwiches," *Reference & User Services Quarterly* 38, no. 1 (1998); Khalid Mahmood and John V. Richardson Jr, "Adoption of Web 2.0 in Us Academic Libraries: A Survey of Arl Library Websites," *Program* 45, no. 4 (2011).

10. Andy Burkhardt, "Social Media: A Guide for College and University Libraries," *College & Research Libraries News* 71, no. 1 (2010); Nancy Davis Kho, "Social Media in Libraries Keys to Deeper Engagement," *Information Today* 28, no. 6 (2011).

11. J. A. Claridge and T. C. Fabian, "History and Development of Evidence-Based Medicine," *World J Surg* 29, no. 5 (2005).

12. L. A. Maggio and J. Y. Kung, "How Are Medical Students Trained to Locate Biomedical Information to Practice Evidence-Based Medicine? A Review of the 2007–2012 Litera-

ture," *J Med Libr Assoc* 102, no. 3 (2014); J. D. Eldredge et al., "Current Practices in Library/ Informatics Instruction in Academic Libraries Serving Medical Schools in the Western United States: A Three-Phase Action Research Study," *BMC Med Educ* 13 (2013); J. L. Dorsch and G. J. Perry, "Evidence-Based Medicine at the Intersection of Research Interests between Academic Health Sciences Librarians and Medical Educators: A Review of the Literature," *J Med Libr Assoc* 100, no. 4 (2012); Lauren A. Maggio, Nancy Durieux, and Nancy H. Tannery, "Librarians in Evidence-Based Medicine Curricula: A Qualitative Study of Librarian Roles, Training, and Desires for Future Development," *Medical Reference Services Quarterly* 34, no. 4 (2015).

13. Kho, "Social Media in Libraries."

14. N. L. Wilczynski and R. B. Haynes, "Response to Corrao et al.: Improving Efficacy of Pubmed Clinical Queries for Retrieving Scientifically Strong Studies on Treatment," *J Am Med Inform Assoc* 14, no. 2 (2007).

15. J. B. Wagner et al., "Three Professions Come Together for an Interdisciplinary Approach to 3d Printing: Occupational Therapy, Biomedical Engineering, and Medical Librarianship," *J Med Libr Assoc* 106, no. 3 (2018).

16. Michelle Dalton, "Key Performance Indicators in Irish Hospital Libraries: Developing Outcome-Based Metrics to Support Advocacy and Service Delivery," *Evidence Based Library and Information Practice* 7, no. 4 (2012).

17. R. Brian et al., "Evaluating the Impact of Clinical Librarians on Clinical Questions During Inpatient Rounds," *J Med Libr Assoc* 106, no. 2 (2018).

18. S. McKeown et al., "Evaluation of Hospital Staff's Perceived Quality of Librarian-Mediated Literature Searching Services," *J Med Libr Assoc* 105 (2017).

19. J. G. Marshall et al., "The Value of Library and Information Services in Patient Care: Results of a Multisite Study," *J Med Libr Assoc* 101, no. 1 (2013).

Chapter Three

Embracing Patient- and Family-Centered Care

A Brief History, Literature Review, and Cross-Walk Analysis with the Joint Commission Standards

Antonio P. DeRosa and Becky Baltich Nelson

WHAT IS PATIENT- AND FAMILY-CENTERED CARE?

Patient- and family-centered care (PFCC) is an evolving concept, generally understood as an approach to patient care that prioritizes the development of partnerships between patients, their families, and health-care providers to ensure that all are involved in decision-making and care. It asks health-care providers to take time to understand each patient and his/her family's values and preferences and to consider health care a collaborative process.[1]

The initial focus on a purposeful incorporation of the patient and their family into health care began in pediatrics. Walking through a pediatric unit in a hospital today, it is common to see parents, siblings, grandparents, and friends at the bedside—comforting the patients, participating in their care, and engaging with the health-care staff; however, this was not always the case. As recently as the mid-twentieth century, parents often had only limited access to their hospitalized children and limited access to information about the care they were receiving.[2] When illness required extended hospital stays, this distance from their families often caused lasting psychological trauma for the patient. This has been termed *hospitalism*, which is the deterioration of a child's health due to extended stays. In the years following World War II, attitudes toward children's well-being started to shift, and new perspectives on childhood development began to emerge.[3] For example, in 1954, the Citizen's Committee on Children in New York City conducted a study to learn more about visiting hours in pediatric units. They found that 60 percent of hospitals (accounting for 72 percent of hospital beds in the city) only allowed visitors three or fewer days per week, often only in one-hour blocks.[4] Their report pointed out that

> it seems reasonable that services for children should be designed with due consideration for that family unit. When a child is sick, his need for the comfort and support of his parents is even greater than usual, and, when he enters the hospital the need can be almost overwhelming. It therefore seems wise that parents should be with their child, to comfort them by their presence and be reassured about his progress.[5]

This is one example of the rising interest in children's health and family involvement in health care, but it is certainly not the first or last. The shift has been gradual and sporadic, with localized initiatives occurring—some sustained some not—in hospitals and clinics around the world. In fact, in reading the literature on PFCC history, one encounters varying timelines filled with diverse examples of activity. Some of these examples discussed below illustrate, but do not exhaust, this history.

In 1965, the Association for the Care of Children's Health was founded to promote the emotional and developmental needs of children and the roles of parents in their care. This group focused on changing the culture of care through education, research, and advocacy; but change happened slowly. Despite its mission to support children and families, the association was hesitant to allow parents to join the organization. The participating heathcare providers worried that the parents' interests would overwhelm their own and they would lose control of the organization.[6] It took thirteen years before parents were permitted to join and work as collaborators.

Similar concerns were shared among other practitioners working in this area. Understanding those concerns, Harvey Picker, founder of the Picker Institute, wanted to "change the fabric of care instead of tinkering at the margins, and he wanted to do it as a friend of the court, not by attacking the health professions."[7] The Picker Institute coined the term *patient-centered care*. Its eight principles were developed from a research project that actively involved patients and families.[8] These principles are:

1. respect for patient's values, preferences, and expressed needs;
2. coordinated and integrated care;
3. clear, high-quality information and education for the patient and family;
4. physical comfort, including pain management;
5. access to care;
6. emotional support to relieve fear and anxiety;
7. involvement of family and friends; and

8. continuity and secure transitions between health care settings.[9]

While patient-centered care may have started with pediatrics, its applicability to all patient types and health-care settings was eventually recognized.

At the forefront of this charge is the Institute for Patient- and Family-Centered Care (IFPCC), founded in 1992 and known until 2010 as the Institute for Patient-Centered Care. The IFPCC hosts national and international conferences, develops educational materials, conducts research, and provides consulting and training sessions—all in an effort to promote the cultural and structural shifts in the provision of health care.[10]

Like the IPFCC, the Institute of Medicine (IOM) also promotes patient- and family-centered care. In a 2001 semi-annual report, *Crossing the Quality Chasm*, the IOM proposed a strategy for redesigning the health-care system. This redesign involved six goals, one of which was patient-centered care. The report defines patient-centered care as "providing care that is respectful of and responsive to individual patient preferences, needs, and values, and ensuring that patient values guide all clinical decisions."[11] Despite advocacy by these and other organizations, to date, a large-scale adoption of patient- and family-centered care has not occurred. To better understand this, the IFPCC identified three main types of barriers to the implementation and practice of PFCC: attitudinal, educational, and organizational barriers.[12] See figure 3.1 for visual representation of the barriers.

Because these barriers to PFCC remain in many health-care settings, patients and their families may still feel excluded from or unable to understand discussions and decisions about their care. When PFCC is standard practice and shared decision-making is the norm, patient satisfaction, adherence to treatment, and practitioner satisfaction increases.[13] PFCC results in lowered health-care costs and utilization of medical resources—including fewer visits to specialty providers, fewer hospitalizations, and fewer laboratory and diagnostic tests.[14] Meeting the needs of patients and their families will require health-care organizations and practitioners to find new and creative ways to overcome barriers in a rapidly changing health-care environment. PFCC can help them do this.

THE CLINICAL MEDICAL LIBRARIAN AND PFCC

Clinical medical librarians (CML) and other health information professionals can and should contribute to PFCC programs in their hospitals, medical schools, or academic medical centers. To evaluate the role CMLs play in PFCC, the remainder of this chapter focuses on the Joint Commission's "Checklist on Advancing Effective Communication, Cultural Competence, and Patient- and Family-Centered Care" report published in 2010. This re-

Attitudinal Barriers

- Fear that patients' and families' suggestions will be unreasonable
- Fear that patients and families will compromise confidentiality
- Belief that a customer service program is sufficient to ensure patient satisfaction and involvement
- Perception that there is a lack of evidence for patient- and family-centered practices
- Belief that patient- and family-centered care is not necessary ("We are knowledgeable, caring professionals. We know what is best for our patients. We are all patients.")
- Belief that patient- and family-centered care is time-consuming and too costly
- Belief that their patients are too poor, too violent, too uneducated, or too humble to be engaged or to engage with their healthcare

Educational Barriers

- Lack of understanding and skills for collaboration on the part of health care professionals and administrators as well as patients and families
- Leaders' lack of understanding of patient- and family-centered care and its benefits
- Organizations unprepared to provide patient and family members with training and support to effectively participate in collaborative endeavors

Organizational Barriers

- Lack of guiding vision
- Tendency to implement either a top-down approach to initiating partnerships with insufficient effort put in to building staff commitment, or tendency to implement a grass-roots effort that lacks leadership commitment and support
- Organizational culture
- Scarce fiscal resources and competing priorities
- Inadequate organizational leadership

Figure 3.1. Potential Barriers to Acceptance and Implementation of Patient- and Family-Centered Care. *Adapted from "Partnering with Patients and Families to Design a Patient- and Family-Centered Health Care System"*

port describes a roadmap for hospitals to assess the unique needs of patients and their caregivers in addition to consideration of clinical aspects of care. The nonclinical needs of patients can range from effective communication, to improving health literacy, and a better understanding of cultural competence. The Joint Commission report provides methods for hospitals to improve their efforts to ensure all patients receive the same level of care regardless of demographics, background, and other socioeconomic characteristics.

Identifying Opportunities for Involvement: A Cross-Walk Analysis

The checklist provided in the Joint Commission report covers all aspects of a patient's continuum of care: admission; assessment; treatment; end-of-life care; discharge and transfer; and organization readiness. Details within each of these steps map to the main principles of PFCC. Using the Institute for Patient- and Family-Centered Care's definition of PFCC, a cross-walk between the Joint Commission's checklist and the core concepts found in the IPFCC definition was reviewed. See table 3.1 for a display of the author's efforts to simplify a cross-walk of the Joint Commission checklist to four PFCC core concepts: (1) dignity and respect; (2) information sharing; (3) participation; and (4) collaboration.

Table 3.1.   Cross-Walk Analysis between Joint Commission Checklist and PFCC Core Concepts

Joint Commission Checklist	PFCC Core Concepts
Admission	
Inform patients of their rights.	Dignity and Respect
Identify the patient's preferred language for discussing health care.	Dignity and Respect
Identify whether the patient has a sensory or communication need.	Dignity and Respect
Determine whether the patient needs assistance completing admission forms.	*Information Sharing*
Collect patient race and ethnicity data in the medical record.	Dignity and Respect
Identify if the patient uses any assistive devices.	Dignity and Respect
Ask the patient if there are any additional needs that may affect his or her care.	Dignity and Respect
Communicate information about unique patient needs that may affect his or her care.	Dignity and Respect
Assessment	
Identify and address patient communication needs during assessment.	Dignity and Respect
Begin the patient-provider relationship with an introduction.	Dignity and Respect
Support the patient's ability to understand and act on health information.	*Information Sharing*
Identify and address patient mobility needs during assessment.	Dignity and Respect
Identify patient cultural, religious, or spiritual beliefs or practices that influence care.	Dignity and Respect
Identify patient dietary needs or restrictions that affect care.	Participation
Ask the patient to identify a support person.	Participation
Communicate information about unique patient needs to the care team.	Dignity and Respect
Treatment	
Address patient communication needs during treatment.	Dignity and Respect

Action	Principle
Monitor changes in the patient's communication status.	Dignity and Respect
Involve patients and families in the care process.	Participation
Tailor the informed consent process to meet patient needs.	*Dignity and Respect; Information Sharing*
Provide patient education that meets patient needs.	*Information Sharing*
Address patient mobility needs during treatment.	Dignity and Respect
Accommodate patient cultural, religious, or spiritual beliefs and practices.	Dignity and Respect
Monitor changes in dietary needs or restrictions that may impact the patient's care.	Participation
Ask the patient to choose a support person if one is not already identified.	Participation
Communicate information about unique patient needs to the care team.	Dignity and Respect

End-of-Life Care

Action	Principle
Address patient communication needs during end-of-life care.	Dignity and Respect
Monitor changes in the patient's communication status during end-of-life care.	Dignity and Respect
Involve the patient's surrogate decision-maker and family in end-of-life care.	*Information Sharing; Participation*
Address patient mobility needs during end-of-life care.	Dignity and Respect
Identify patient cultural, religious, or spiritual beliefs and practices at the end of life.	Dignity and Respect
Make sure the patient has access to his or her chosen support person.	Participation

Discharge and Transfer

Action	Principle
Address patient communication needs during discharge and transfer.	Dignity and Respect
Engage patient and families in discharge and transfer planning and instruction.	Participation
Provide discharge instruction that meets patient needs.	*Information Sharing*

Identify follow-up providers that can meet unique patient needs.	Dignity and Respect; Participation; Collaboration;
Organization Readiness	
Create an environment that is inclusive of all patients.	Dignity and Respect; Collaboration
Develop a system to provide language services.	Dignity and Respect; Collaboration
Address the communication needs of patients with sensory or communication impairments.	Dignity and Respect; Collaboration
Integrate health literacy strategies into patient discussions and materials.	*Information Sharing; Collaboration*
Incorporate cultural competence and patient- and family-centered care concepts into care delivery.	Dignity and Respect; Collaboration

Elements coded as "Information Sharing" are italicized.

The authors focus on the IPFCC core concept of "information sharing" to present examples from the literature of current CML contributions to PFCC programming in their hospitals. The subcategories of leadership; data collection and use; workforce; and patient, family, and community engagement that fall under the "organization readiness" group of the checklist are omitted from the analysis in this chapter because they are out of scope and unrelated to the "information sharing" concept—which is most aligned with the work of CMLs.

By assessing the crosswalk analysis, the Joint Commission checklist items coded as "information sharing" are synthesized into three main themes: (1) contributing to improved health literacy levels of patients; (2) ensuring patient education materials are written at an appropriate literacy and reading level; and (3) informational support for caregivers and surrogate decision-makers. Combining the major terms and phrases in these themes with librarian and information professional terminology, the authors devised the following comprehensive search strategy in MEDLINE to scope the literature on any PFCC programs in which librarians are participating: *((("health literacy" OR "patient education" OR "caregiver support" OR "caregiver education" OR "reading level" OR "reading levels" OR "information support" OR "informational support" OR "patient needs" OR "education materials" OR "educational materials" OR "literacy level" OR "literacy levels" OR "literacy needs" OR "reading needs" OR "Health Literacy"[Mesh] OR "Patient Education as Topic"[Mesh])) AND ((librarian OR librarians OR informationist OR informationists OR "information professionals" OR "information specialist" OR "information specialists" OR "Librarians"[Mesh]))*. A review of the literature follows.

To tackle the first "information sharing" theme of the cross-walk above, CMLs and other information professionals are contributing to the health literacy of patients in several ways. Shipman et al. describe the development of a curriculum to educate health providers and medical staff on health literacy principles in an effort to improve the patient experience and understanding of care.[15] In two separate research studies, Tarver et al. detail the process of setting up MedlinePlus Connect in an institution's electronic medical record (EMR) system, Epic, to allow for seamless inclusion of contextual information and development of a search box linking patients to MedlinePlus within the patient portal. This included training sessions for staff and patients on using MedlinePlus and accessing trusted health information online.[16] Tarver et al. also published a 2016 case report on creating a comic book to educate children in an effort to improve their knowledge of obesity and increase their health literacy levels.[17] Grabeel et al. and Six-Means provide examples of how collaborating with nurses and other health professionals can lead to the perception of librarians as thought-leaders and advocates for health literacy education among patients. Grabeel et al. collaborated with key university medical center providers to create a web-based patient education clearinghouse consisting of in-house and other vetted materials written in plain language available for download from Epic to share with patients at the point of care.[18] Grabeel et al. collaborated with patient education champions and nurses to survey the health literacy landscape at a university medical center. Survey results led to staff training by librarians who were viewed as the experts in health literacy instruction.[19] DeRosa et al. and Oelschlegel et al. use their patient resource centers and health information centers (respectively) to offer health-literacy-related and educational programming to patients. DeRosa et al. holds regular health education seminars on a number of medical topics to improve the knowledge base of their patient populations.[20] These seminars allow the consumer health librarians to assess health literacy levels of seminar attendees in order to provide targeted and appropriate information. Oelschlegel et al. detail the steps taken to develop patient programming in their health information center to combat low health literacy among their patient population.[21] Finally, Raimondo et al. devised a service to help campus researchers use best practices in health communication with human subjects where librarians teach health literacy workshops and provide a consent form review service for principal investigators.[22]

The next "information sharing" theme surrounding patient education materials derived from the crosswalk analysis addresses a different set of CML skills. Zipperer et al. and McMullen et al. describe instructional programs developed to train practitioners on consumer health resources and to help them understand the unique information needs of patients. Zipperer et al. present a survey analysis of the library community's role in the information dimensions of patient safety.[23] Findings and examples include developing educational resource guides and training staff to increase their skills in patient safety. McMullen et al. describe outreach efforts to improve the patient-education programming in a matrix of free clinics affiliated with their university medical center.[24] Librarians employ a "train the trainer" approach to expanding instruction on MedlinePlus and other consumer health resources to, in turn, be offered and taught to patients. Lindner et al. explain the process of making patient-education rounds on nursing units in their medical center.[25] Through direct patient consultation and assessment of information needs, librarians provide just-in-time information to patients and their families to supplement care plans and increase the knowledge of medical conditions/treatments. Lastly, Klein-Fedyshin et al. discuss ways that the specialized curation skills of librarians lead to patients' understanding of care and empower their decision-making.[26] By selecting and providing targeted educational videos to accompany textual information and materials, librarians allow patients to digest information on their own time and at their own pace from the comfort of their homes. Patients are better able to retain information related to their care as a result of this.

The third "information sharing" theme of CML support for caregivers and surrogate decision-makers is less represented in the literature than the two previous themes. A commentary published in the *Journal of the Medical Library Association* calls for health sciences librarians to provide better outreach to family caregivers of patients. Howrey provides examples of strategies librarians can take to reach this underserved, yet critical, population of the health-care system—advocacy for caregiving public policy, resource-building, programming, and education.[27] This framework could provide a roadmap for CMLs to better reach and support the information needs of patient decision partners/proxies. Perhaps a more concrete example of reaching caregivers is a case study presented by Flewelling on library outreach to support groups.[28] Oftentimes, caregivers and families of patients attend support group meetings, an effective venue for introducing the role of librarians to provide information on a patient's case to help surrogate decision-makers choose the best course of treatment for a loved one. By presenting to key support groups and focusing on information services tailored to their unique needs, librarians can help caregivers be more informed to make confident and empowered decisions.

The PFCC model, a disruptor to traditional medicine, will undoubtedly take time to be fully implemented. Influence from within health-care professions and payment sources, like Medicare and insurance companies, will aid in the transition; however, the real contribution will come from those on the ground. Patients and their families need to be more active in their health care, and providers need to engage with patients and focus on creating meaningful collaborative relationships. Both groups require support and tools librarians can provide.

NOTES

1. Aaron M. Clay and Bridget Parsh, "Patient- and Family-Centered Care: It's Not Just for Pediatrics Anymore," *AMA Journal of Ethics* 18, no. 1 (2016): 40–44. doi:10.1001/journalofethics.2016.18.1.medu3-1601.

2. Nora Wells, "Historical Perspective on Family-Centered Care," *Acad Pediatr* 11, no. 2 (2011): 100–102 (2011). doi:10.1016/j.acap.2011.01.007.

3. Jeremy Jolley and Linda Shields, "The Evolution of Family-Centered Care," *J Pediatr Nurs* 24, no. 2 (2009): 164–70. doi:10.1016/j.pedn.2008.03.010.

4. Citizen's Committee on Children in New York City, "LIBERAL Visiting Policies for Children in Hospitals," *J Pediatr* 46, no. 6 (1995): 710–16.

5. Citizen's Committee on Children in New York City, "LIBERAL Visiting Policies for Children in Hospitals."

6. Beverly H. Johnson, "The Changing Role of Families in Health Care," *Children's Health Care: J Assoc Care Child Health* 19, no. 4 (1990): 234–41. doi:10.1207/s15326888chc1904_7.

7. D. F. Beatrice, C. P. Thomas, and B. Biles, "Grant Making with an Impact: The Picker/Commonwealth Patient-Centered Care Program," *Health Aff (Project Hope)* 17, no. 1 (1998): 236–44.

8. Michael J. Barry and Susan Edgman-Levitan, "Shared Decision Making—Pinnacle of Patient-Centered Care," *NEJM* 366, no. 9 (2012): 780–81. doi:10.1056/NEJMp1109283.

9. James V. Rawson and Julie Moretz, "Patient- and Family-Centered Care: A Primer," *J AM Coll Radiol* 13, no. 12 pt. B (2016): 1544–49. doi:10.1016/j.jacr.2016.09.003.

10. B. H. Johnson and M. R. Abraham, *Partnering with Patients, Residents, and Families: A Resource for Leaders of Hospitals, Ambulatory Care Settings, and Long-Term Care Communities* (Bethesda, MD: Institute for Patient-and Family-Centered Care, 2012).

11. A. Wolfe, "Institute of Medicine Report: Crossing the Quality Chasm: A New Health Care System for the 21st Century," *Policy, Politics, & Nursing Practice* 2, no. 3 (2001): 233–35. doi:10.1177/152715440100200312.

12. J. Conway, B. Johnson, and S. Edgman-Levitan, "Partnering with Patients and Families to Design a Patient- and Family-Centered Health Care System: A Roadmap for the Future: A Work in Progress," *Family-Centered Care* (2006).

13. The Joint Commission, *Advancing Effective Communication, Cultural Competence, and Patient- and Family-Centered Care: A Roadmap for Hospitals* (Oakbrook Terrace, IL: The Joint Commission, 2010).

14. Klea D. Bertakis and Rahman Azari, "Patient-Centered Care Is Associated with Decreased Health Care Utilization," *J Am Board Fam Med* 24, no. 3 (2011): 229–39. doi:10.3122/jabfm.2011.03.100170.

15. Jean P. Shipman, Sabrina Kurtz-Rossi, and Carla J. Funk, "The Health Information Literacy Research Project," *JMLA* 97, no. 4 (2009): 293–301. doi:10.3163/1536-5050.97.4.014.

16. Talicia Tarver, Dixie A. Jones, Mararia Adams, and Alejandro Garcia, "The Librarian's Role in Linking Patients to Their Personal Health Data and Contextual Information," *Med Ref Serv Q* 32, no. 4 (2013): 459–67. doi:10.1080/02763869.2013.837730.

17. Talicia Tarver et al., "A Novel Tool for Health Literacy: Using Comic Books to Combat Childhood Obesity," *J Hosp Librariansh* 16, no. 2 (2016): 152–59. doi:10.1080/15323269.2016.1154768.

18. Amy Six-Means, "Health Literacy's Influence on Consumer Libraries," *Med Ref Serv Q* 36, no. 1 (2017): 79–89. doi:10.1080/02763869.2017.1259920.

19. Kelsey L. Grabeel and Cynthia J Beeler, "Taking the Pulse of the University of Tennessee Medical Center's Health Literacy Knowledge," *Med Ref Serv Q* 37, no. 1 (2018): 89–96. doi:10.1080/02763869.2017.1404399.

20. Antonio P. DeRosa and Judy C. Stribling, "A Case Report of Health Seminars Supporting Patient Education, Engagement, and Health Literacy," *J Consum Health Internet* 22, no. 3 (2018): 238–43. doi:10.1080/15398285.2018.1513269.

21. Sandy Oelschlegel et al., "Librarians Promoting Changes in the Health Care Delivery System through Systematic Assessment," *Med Ref Serv Q* 37, no. 2 (2018): 142–52. doi:10.1080/02763869.2018.1439216.

22. Paula G. Raimondo, Ryan L. Harris, Michele Nance, and Everly D. Brown, "Health Literacy and Consent Forms: Librarians Support Research on Human Subjects," *JMLA* 102, no. 1 (2014): 5–8. doi:10.3163/1536-5050.102.1.003.

23. Lorri Zipperer and Jan Sykes, "The Role of Librarians in Patient Safety: Gaps and Strengths in the Current Culture," *JMLA* 92, no. 4 (2004): 498–500.

24. Karen D. McMullen, Rozalynd P. McConnaughy, and Ruth A. Riley, "Outreach to Improve Patient Education at South Carolina Free Medical Clinics," *J Consum Health Internet* 15, no. 2 (2011): 117–31. doi:10.1080/15398285.2011.572779.

25. Katherine L. Lindner and Lia Sabbagh, "In a New Element: Medical Librarians Making Patient Education Rounds," *JMLA* 92, no. 1 (2004): 94–97.

26. Michele Klein-Fedyshin, Michelle L. Burda, Barbara A. Epstein, and Barbara Lawrence, "Collaborating to Enhance Patient Education and Recovery," *JMLA* 93, no. 4 (2005): 440–45.

27. Mary M. Howrey, "Health Sciences Library Outreach to Family Caregivers: A Call to Service," *JMLA* 106, no. 2 (2018): 251–58. doi:10.5195/jmla.2018.390.

28. Kate W. Flewelling, "Library Outreach to Support Groups: A Case Study," *J Hosp Librariansh* 9, no. 4 (2009): 362–71. doi:10.1080/15323260903251922.

Chapter Four

Consumer Information Therapy on Pediatric Rounds

Judy C. Stribling

This chapter describes and discusses the role of librarians in patient-centered care (PCC), health literacy, and the activities of a team of clinical medical librarians who practice PCC by conducting consumer rounds and delivering health information directly to hospitalized patients/caregivers in a pediatric clinical department at a large academic medical center.

The evolving role of clinical medical librarians is well chronicled in literature.[1] Librarians involved in clinical work owe a debt of gratitude to Gertrude Lamb's groundbreaking program established at the University of Missouri–Kansas City School of Medicine in 1971.[2] Lamb's discernment of clinicians' information needs and foresight in building a service program to address those needs was genius:

> to provide information quickly to physicians and other members of the health care team; to influence the information-seeking behavior of clinicians and improve their library skills; and to establish the medical librarian's role as a valid member of the health care team.[3]

The practice of providing health information to patients gained slower traction in the professional library world, although McKnight's historical review of "physician-ordered reading for patients—sometimes facilitated by a librarian" reveals a long history and recognition of the need for "bibliotherapy."[4] As PCC, the process of including patients/caregivers in clinical care decisions [5] becomes normative, the role of the librarian (clinical or consumer health) in PCC can and should be more fully realized and opportunities for more involvement explored.

Lee et al. discuss numerous issues that searching for health information on the internet may cause for patients/caregivers. These include becoming overloaded with information, misunderstanding technical language, and discovering irrelevant or misleading results.[6] Misinformation can easily lead to incorrect self-diagnoses of chronic or fatal diseases. When conducting health research on behalf of self, family, or other loves ones, even the most well-trained information professional can become confused by the large volume of data and conflicting information. Patients/caregivers lacking the search and appraisal skills of a medical librarian are more likely to discover dubious results. Yet many amateur searchers believe even simple internet search results adequately address their health information needs.[7] Physicians in emergency departments report that almost 25 percent of their patients arrive with an internet-based self-diagnosis.[8]

Diagnosing a health condition is complicated, and a diagnosis is merely the starting point for patient/caregiver questions. Follow-up questions multiply and lead many patients/caregivers further toward internet search engines, where results are based on multiple advertisement and popularity algorithms.[9] Complex medical terminology or mixed messages from disparate resources can lead to increased anxiety for patients/caregivers.[10] What is the best treatment for what I have? What are my chances for total recovery? How will this medicine affect me, and do I really need this test? Will he ever remember me again, and how do I keep him from wandering out of the neighborhood? Health-care providers, often pressed to see more patients in less time, do not have the bandwidth to answer all questions for patients/caregivers.

While health-care providers may not be the most effective literacy communicators, librarians are almost ideally suited for the job.[11] Medical librarians with specialized consumer health training are taught to recognize when patients/caregivers may need additional information assistance. Six-Means suggests, "Librarians need to help patrons realize their specific information needs and to be a resource, both at that moment and in the future."[12]

HEALTH LITERACY

Health literacy, "the ability to obtain, process, and understand basic health information and services needed to make appropriate health decisions,"[13] is an important skill for building healthy people and communities. In the United States, low health literacy is a national problem; over 80 million adults have basic or below health literacy skills.[14] Low health literacy puts patients at greater risk for limited access to care and poorer outcomes, and places a serious strain on our medical system.

Low health literacy has special detrimental implications for children because they depend on parents and caregivers to help make treatment decisions.[15] Health literacy, similar to information literacy, requires people of all ages and educational levels to acquire additional skills such as information-seeking behavior.[16] Information therapy to raise health literacy increases the chance for better patient outcomes.[17] Raising health literacy is a dynamic issue requiring system-level changes for health professionals and organizations.[18]

Inpatient Setting

People are more likely to ask questions when they are informed, empowered, and confident. There are fewer places where one feels more vulnerable and powerless than a hospital bed. Essential patient information needs may not be addressed during bedside rounds, despite the close interactions between the health-care team and the patient/caregiver.[19] Relying heavily on nursing staff and medical residents to deliver health information and education to them, some patients/caregivers may not want to ask for information because of embarrassment of their diagnosis or symptoms or believe that clinical staff is overworked and too busy to answer questions.

Librarians can address information needs by rounding on floors and teaching patients/caregivers where to look for reliable online health resources and helping them evaluate the results. Information delivery to patients/caregivers by medical librarians is a value-added service for everyone involved. Physicians trust clinical medical librarians to deliver appropriate information, and patients/caregivers are grateful to receive the information.

CASE STUDY PEDIATRIC ROUNDING

Clinical medical librarians at Weill Cornell Medicine (WCM), Samuel J. Wood Library (Wood Library) began providing information therapy to patients, families, and caregivers on the Phyllis and David Komansky Center for Children's Health pediatric floors of New York-Presbyterian Hospital (NYP) in August 2016, by conducting twice-weekly patient rounds.[20] WCM librarians and clinicians in the Department of Pediatrics at NYP enjoy a long-standing working relationship; librarians participate in weekly clinical rounds with attendings and residents and teach evidence-based medicine to first-year medical students and those in third-year pediatric clinical rotations, as well as to new fellows and residents, including visiting residents from Weill Cornell's Tanzanian affiliate. At least one clinical librarian also attends weekly rounds in the Pediatric Intensive Care Unit (PICU), with the PICU Integrative Medicine and Pediatric Gastroenterology teams.

WCM librarians recognized the time and attention pediatricians, pediatric nurses, and the Child Life staff devoted to educating individual patients/ caregivers during clinical rounding sessions. The education needs of each patient/caregiver are unique, and some require more assistance than others do. Recognizing this, WCM librarians proposed a plan to increase PCC in- itiatives and reduce some of the education load carried by clinicians by visiting hospitalized pediatric patients/caregivers, conducting reference inter- views, researching literature, and delivering consumer health information to the bedside. Librarians utilized a four-component plan to determine pediatric patient/caregiver needs: (1) assess the situation, (2) devise an educational intervention, (3) deliver the intervention, and (4) document educational inter- vention. Assessment considerations included patient/caregiver's preferred language, cultural or religious beliefs about health care and illness, emotional status, and motivation to learn. Mode of intervention and delivery were de- termined during initial assessment.

Design and Planning

The assistant director of clinical library services (assistant director) at Wood Library met with the Department of Pediatrics' chair of quality and patient safety (chair) to establish expectations, identify requirements, and develop a workflow for clinical librarian activity on the patient floors. Development of what became the Pediatric Clinical Library Services (PCLS) program began by identifying team members: associate director of user support, research and education of Wood Library, the assistant director, two clinical medical librar- ians (CMLs), and a clinical medical library intern (intern). PCLS team mem- bers must be HIPAA certified, up to date on vaccinations required by NYP, and aware of Joint Commission standards.

The five-member team defined the program's mission and goals, iden- tified key clinical stakeholders—physicians, nurses, social workers, and the hospital's Child Life staff—and drafted an initial service overview. Provid- ing pediatric patients and their family members or caregivers access to reli- able, targeted, and timely health information resources that encourage and enable informed decision-making is the primary function of the PCLS. Im- proving patient/caregiver satisfaction and comfort during their hospital stay, returning health information on the same day requested, and reinforcing the message "Amazing Things Are Happening for Kids" at NYP are included in goals of the PCLS team.

After the goals and services were identified, the PCLS team asked the chair to introduce the new service to other clinical stakeholders within the pediatric department. The chair arranged meetings between the PCLS team and the division chief of clinical pediatrics (chief), patient care directors

(PCDs) from the General Pediatric Unit (Peds), the PICU, and the Neonatal Intensive Care Unit (NICU).

Implementation

PCLS members attend clinical rounds with two different pediatric teams—red or blue—each Tuesday morning and perform consumer rounds on Tuesdays and Thursdays during the "quiet hour" between 1:00 and 2:00 p.m. when clinical activities are at a lull. After Tuesday clinical rounds, informed by information garnered during the morning clinical rounds, the PCLS team distributes appropriate information therapy to patients/caregivers and documents education intervention. On Thursday rounds, PCLS librarians check in at the nursing station to determine if any patients/caregivers on unit have raised specific information needs. PCLS team members also ask if the nurses have evidence-based practice questions and encourage them to utilize the librarians' skills and resources.

Patients/caregivers with known information therapy needs, determined either from direct patient/caregiver or from health-care provider requests, receive immediate attention. Otherwise, the team rounds, visiting every room unless the patient is clearly at rest or receiving a clinical procedure. Upon entering a patient's room, the team engages with both the patient and present family members by loosely following the script below:

> Hello, we just wanted to take a minute of your time to introduce ourselves: My name is _____ and this is _____. We are consumer health librarians.
> We help patients and their families get health information that is easy to read and understand and trust. It can be information about your current diagnosis, treatment, or any other health or wellness questions you might have.

Rounding procedures in the PICU are different from general Peds for a number of reasons. PICU patients are critically ill, the unit has no official quiet time, and rooms contain multiple beds with an individual nursing station positioned at the entrance of each room. The team checks in with nurses at each station unless it appears a patient is in crisis or a clinical procedure is in process. Nurses refer PCLS team members to patients or families they think may have information needs and to those whose health status is stable enough for a visit. PICU nurses are also encouraged to ask evidence-based practice questions at this time. Providing research support to nurses is highly valued, especially at hospitals seeking Magnet status.

All patient education interventions are recorded on a HIPAA-compliant request log with no identifying patient data other than room number to track patient information inquiries. The form contains fields for the date of information request, room number, patient's questions, information medium or delivery method, and a field to note questions answered and information delivered. To maintain privacy, the forms remain in a locked drawer in the assistant director's office.

Information Sources and Patient Preferences

Assessing the health literacy of patients/caregivers and appreciating cultural preferences is of prime importance when planning health interventions. Assessments consider preferred language, cultural, or religious beliefs about health care and illness, emotional status of patients/caregivers, and their desire or motivation to learn. Professional patient-care staff must assess and document patient and family educational needs and incorporate the information into a care plan. Librarians are uniquely poised to assist the medical team in this responsibility.

PCLS librarians consult a variety of sources to answer consumer health questions. The most common resources are: Access Pediatrics, Clinical Key Patient Education, Medline Plus, MICROMEDEX Care Notes, and UpTo-Date Patient Education resources. PCLS team members search for the most appropriate pediatric consumer health information to share with patients. All patients/caregivers are educated on how to find reliable health information on the internet and are given a copy of the National Library of Medicine's MedLinePlus brochure.

The number of clinical trials carried out in children is relatively few worldwide due to ethical concerns about inclusion of children in clinical trials.[21] There are significant gaps in pediatric health research and scientific literature, which affect the availability of appropriate consumer health information. When pediatric-specific information for a patient or parent's question is unavailable, PCLS librarians create a summary of evidence from the best available health resources.

Patients may opt to have information delivered by print at bedside, by email, or by U.S. mail. PCLS team members make every effort to deliver information the same day but no later than twenty-four hours from request. PCLS team members respect the privacy and confidence of all patient inquiries. If a patient asks questions that may affect a clinical care plan, librarians ask for the patient's permission to share the request with the clinical care team.

Three-Month Assessment

The PCLS team benchmarked pediatric information therapy interactions during the first three months of service. Between August 9 and October 27, 2016, the PCLS team conducted twenty-four rounds on the general Peds and PICU floors, answered ninety-four patient, family, or health-provider questions, and delivered 139 health information items in a variety of formats.

Although a majority of patients/caregivers requested hardcopies of the information, a few viewed MedLinePlus tutorial videos. Information therapy requests fell into five broad categories: (1) where to go online to find valuable health information, (2) how to find out more about my diagnosis, (3) what are the side effects of my medication, (4) I want to know more details about the procedure I am going to have, and (5) what do I need to know when I leave the hospital.

Anecdotal evidence suggested the PCLS program satisfied the needs of patients' family members. One mother, concerned about her twelve-year-old son receiving narcotic pain medication, asked PCLS team members about pediatric morphine dosing. When asked if the information she received was informative, she replied, "Yes, it was very helpful. I wasn't happy about him having to take that medication, but if he needs it, I'm OK. I feel much better about it now." Team librarians develop familiarity with patients requiring long or repeated hospital stays. One long-stay patient's mother relied heavily on the PCLS team to augment information about her son's difficult diagnosis and credited the librarians for "making us all feel a little more in control." Told he could contact the PCLS team after hospital discharge, a father said, "For parents at home, information is everything. This is great."

Clinicians appeared equally pleased with services provided by the librarians. The PCD of the PICU wrote to the Weill Cornell Medicine Library Director about the program, "Parents and staff have been thoroughly impressed with the service offered by the librarian team and very appreciative of the information they have provided. I am looking forward to working with them on evidence-based nursing quality improvement projects. Thank you for offering such a great service for our families and staff." Other nurses have commented: "What a wonderful service; this will be very helpful"; "Awesome idea!"; and "I'm calling on you when I do my EBP project."

EMR Access

At the two-year mark of the program, the assistant director met with the chief to request access to the electronic medical record (EMR) for the PCLS team. The chief agreed PCLS team education interventions were valuable and warranted documentation in the patient's medical record. She discussed privacy issues related to giving PCLS members access to the EMRs with her technical, legal, and medical team. After securing approval, the chief asked NYP's Information Technology Team (NYP IT) to design a unique note field in the EMR for members of the PCLS to record education interventions with patients/caregivers. This privilege enabled librarians to better meet information needs and raised the status of the team's responsibilities and duties.

Before accessing the EMR, PCLS members achieved certificates of completion in all modules of a proprietary clinical training program. Modules within the program address Joint Commission standards such as the environment of care, infection prevention and control, provision of care, national patient safety goals, privacy and information security compliance, annual hospital topics for providers, worker safety, impaired health-care workers and drug diversion, and fire safety training.

The PCLS team designed a new workflow for documenting interactions using the EMR and were able to retire the former paper-based log (figure 4.1).

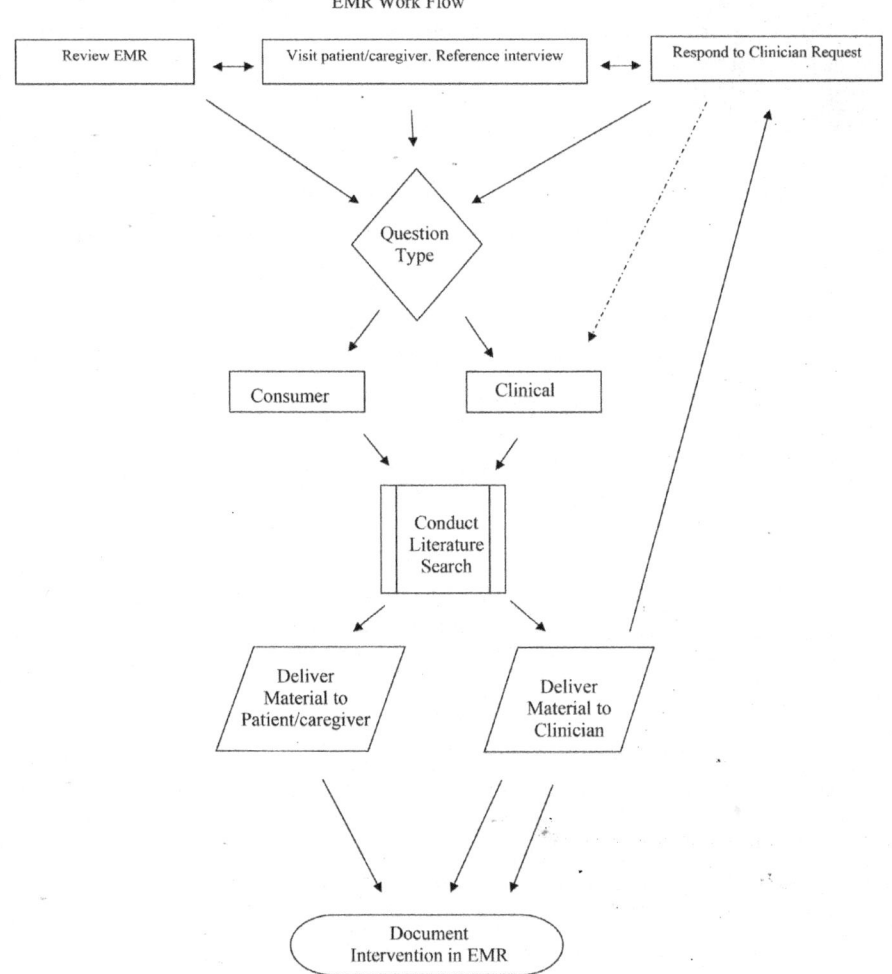

Figure 4.1.   Documenting Interactions Using the EMR

Challenges and Discussion

Our experiences developing the consumer pediatric program provide useful lessons for librarians and health-care providers considering a similar project. The author recognizes pediatric units possess distinct policies and cultures, and the PCLS program was tailored for a very specific microclimate at NYP. Although the PCLS program may not be generalizable in whole to other pediatric hospitals, the success of the program was strong enough to encourage librarians at other institutions interested in pediatric patient rounding to engage with physicians, nurses, and (when applicable) Child Life specialists to develop similar services.

Working with institutional IT departments is critical for success. The most challenging aspect of this project was gaining NYP IT identities for WCM librarians. Although not technically difficult, gaining hospital EMR access for the librarians was challenging and required the assistance of high-level administrators as well as IT technicians. Without a pre-defined process for establishing WCM library identities in the hospital EMR, access was delayed for weeks after permission was granted. Library and hospital administrators should consider this before initiating a similar program.

Interaction between professional librarians and patients/caregivers in clinical environments increases opportunities to assess patient/caregiver information needs and health literacy levels. Receiving medical information support during treatment may improve patient outcomes and comforts patients/caregivers. The business of health care is shifting toward PCC models.[22] Innovative librarians must successfully align existing programs and services in this direction. The service-centered nature of our profession suggests this will not be a hard lift.

NOTES

1. V. Algermissen, "Biomedical Librarians in a Patient Care Setting at the University of Missouri-Kansas City School of Medicine," *Bulletin of the Medical Library Association* 62, no. 4 (1974); K. Cimpl, "Clinical Medical Librarianship: A Review of the Literature," *Bull Med Libr Assoc* 73, no. 1 (1985).

2. C. E. Lipscomb, "Clinical Librarianship," *Bull Med Libr Assoc* 88, no. 4 (2000).

3. Lipscomb, "Clinical Librarianship."

4. Cimpl, "Clinical Medical Librarianship."

5. Michelynn McKnight, "Information Prescriptions, 1930–2013: An International History and Comprehensive Review," *JMLA* 102, no. 4 (2014).

6. B. H. Johnson and M. R. Abraham, *Partnering with Patients, Residents, and Families: A Resource for Leaders of Hospitals, Ambulatory Care Settings, and Long-Term Care Communities* (Bethesda, MD: Institute for Patient-and Family-Centered Care, 2012).

7. B. Bibel, "A New Prescription for Health and Medical Information," *Booklist* 109, no. 7 (2012).

8. D. M. McCarthy et al., "What Did You Google? Describing Online Health Information Search Patterns of Ed Patients and Their Relationship with Final Diagnoses," *West J Emerg Med* 18, no. 5 (2017).

9. K. S. Shuyler and K. M. Knight, "What Are Patients Seeking When They Turn to the Internet? Qualitative Content Analysis of Questions Asked by Visitors to an Orthopaedics Web Site," *J Med Internet Res* 5, no. 4 (2003).

10. E. Anderson, G. Johnson, and L. A. Thomas, "Do Internet Searches Prior to a Doctor Visit Improve Quality and Reduce Costs?" *Int J Health Econo Dev* 4, no. 1 (2018).

11. J. F. Ha and N. Longnecker, "Doctor-Patient Communication: A Review," *Ochsner J* 10, no. 1 (2010); J. P. Shipman, E. Lake, and A. I. Weber, "Improving Health Literacy: Health Sciences Library Case Studies," *Ref Serv Rev* 44, no. 2 (2016).

12. A. Six-Means et al., "Building a Foundation of Health Literacy with Ask Me 3™," *J Consum Health Internet* 16, no. 2 (2012).

13. N. D. Berkman, T. C. Davis, and L. McCormack, "Health Literacy: What Is It?" *Journal Health Commun* 15, no. supplement 2 (2010).

14. M. Kutner et al., *The Health Literacy of America's Adults: Results from the 2003 National Assessment of Adult Literacy* (2006).

15. R. D. Gebhard et al., "Improving Health Literacy: Use of an Informational Brochure Improves Parents' Understanding of Their Child's Fluoroscopic Examination," *AJR Am J Roentgenol* 204, no. 1 (2015).

16. R. L. Rothman et al., "Health Literacy and Quality: Focus on Chronic Illness Care and Patient Safety," *Pediatrics* 124, supplement 3 (2009).

17. N. D. Berkman et al., "Health Literacy Interventions and Outcomes: An Updated Systematic Review," *Evid Rep Technol Assess (Full Rep)*, no. 199 (2011).

18. H. K. Koh et al., "New Federal Policy Initiatives to Boost Health Literacy Can Help the Nation Move Beyond the Cycle of Costly 'Crisis Care,'" *Health Aff (Millwood)* 31, no. 2 (2012); R. W. Batterham et al., "Health Literacy: Applying Current Concepts to Improve Health Services and Reduce Health Inequalities," *Public Health* 132 (2016).

19. S. J. Gentles, C. Lokker, and K. A. McKibbon, "Health Information Technology to Facilitate Communication Involving Health Care Providers, Caregivers, and Pediatric Patients: A Scoping Review," *J Med Internet Res* 12, no. 2 (2010).

20. J. C. Stribling, K. C. Mages, and D. Delgado, "Patient-Centered Rounding in an Inpatient Pediatric Setting," *J Hosp Librariansh* 17, no. 2 (2017).

21. Education Department of Health, "The Belmont Report. Ethical Principles and Guidelines for the Protection of Human Subjects of Research," *J Am Coll Dent* 81, no. 3 (2014).

22. O. Bhattacharyya et al., "Redesigning Care: Adapting New Improvement Methods to Achieve Person-Centred Care," *BMJ Qual Saf* 28, no. 3 (2019).

Chapter Five

Diagnosing and Treating the Patient's Information Needs

A Librarian Provides Information Therapy Using the EMR in an Oncology Setting

Antonio P. DeRosa

THE LIBRARIAN AS CLINICIAN

Are medical librarians clinicians? By definition clinicians hold advanced degrees, knowledge, licenses, and expertise in a medical or health discipline and use their expertise to diagnose and treat patients.[1] Librarians working in hospitals and academic medical centers generally earned graduate degrees (many in both information and library sciences as well as other master's degrees) and have advanced certification in focused health information disciplines such as from the Academy of Health Information Professionals (AHIP) or Consumer Health Information Specializations from the Medical Library Association. Continuing education and extensive training in information resources enable medical librarians to meet patient needs for quality information to help them understand their care and make important treatment decisions.

A well-trained medical librarian with proven skills and experience is an excellent clinical partner and ideally suited for patient-facing roles. Patients and their caregivers (patients/caregivers) need and deserve to more fully comprehend the medical care they are receiving.[2] Possessing targeted information at the right time can lead to patient/caregiver confidence regarding specific medical care, empower patient/caregiver communication with their providers, increase psychological support for treatment decisions, and improve health outcomes.[3] By directly interfacing with patients/caregivers and

53

providers, clinical librarians can diagnose and triage information needs of patients, their loved ones, and other clinical providers.

This chapter describes the experiences and methodologies of an oncology consumer health librarian (OCHL) working in the field as a clinical team member in oncology supportive care services at a world-famous academic medical center.

THE ONCOLOGY CONSUMER HEALTH LIBRARIAN ROLE

The role of the OCHL at Weill Cornell Medicine/New York–Presbyterian Hospital (WCM/NYP) was born from the desire to create patient-centered information and education support for the oncology population in the cancer center. The OCHL was hired to serve as a navigator for patients/caregivers seeking information on medical care or other supportive and clinic services available to them at WCM/NYP. Hospital and cancer center leadership realized the benefits and importance of providing the OCHL with electronic medical record (EMR) privileges. This invaluable access to patient records supports, and makes possible, the success of the OCHL to responsibly provide validated, timely, and accurate information to patients/caregivers based on full knowledge of unique diagnoses, individual treatment, and assessment plans and other clinical considerations.

Dr. David M. Nanus, MD, Mark W. Pasmantier professor of hematology and oncology in medicine and the chief of the Division of Hematology and Medical Oncology at Weill Cornell Medicine, describes the catalyst for creating the OCHL role on the clinical team:

> A diagnosis of cancer is overwhelming for most patients and their families. In addition to coping with the emotional stress and the immediate impact on daily living, patients, families and caregivers must struggle to understand the specific cancer diagnosis and the various treatment options available. In today's oncologic universe, shared decision making between physicians and patients is becoming more the norm than the exception. Where does the patient and his/her family turn to for help and a better understanding? At WCM and NYP, we have an information professional specifically trained in oncology information resources as an invaluable resource for patients and their families to support their decision-making, understanding of care, communication with the care team, and self-advocacy. By providing targeted information therapy to our patients, the Oncology Consumer Health Librarian (OCHL) role supports the clinical and supportive care teams by acting as a resource for patients' and caregivers' information, health literacy, and educational needs. The OCHL works with the physician and the cancer care team to provide in-depth information services specifically for a patient and caregiver based on their diagnosis and medical situation, satisfying their specific needs. This resource is invaluable and welcome by patients, families and the cancer care team. [4]

The primary responsibility of the OCHL is meeting health information needs of the oncology population while promoting consumer-focused research and health literacy programming to patients/caregivers and providers. Research indicates informed patients enjoy more positive health outcomes.[5] Patients with higher literacy levels understand more about their health care and are more likely to communicate and actively participate with providers in the delivery of their care.[6] The OCHL supports a culture of patient- and family-centered care by reviewing patients' charts, scheduling information therapy appointments with these patients, and providing information as well as educating them to find health information related to their care. The OCHL also addresses the serious public health problem of patients who do not feel knowledgeable and confident enough to make informed decisions about their care or communicate openly with their care team.[7]

The OCHL can alleviate some of the patient/caregiver stresses that accompany researching cancer topics by providing information therapy to them about their diagnosis and answering treatment questions. Information therapy helps put patients/caregivers at ease, elicits informed questions for the patient/caregiver to ask their provider(s), facilitates dialogue between patient/caregiver and provider regarding care, and empowers patients/caregivers to make difficult treatment decisions. The OCHL refers patients/caregivers to reputable resources for health and medical information; provides appropriate literacy level, science-based, and consumer health literature to patients/caregivers; and documents these encounters with providers through the EMR. Ideally, the OCHL improves overall patient experience and quality of life during difficult health crises.

DESIGN AND PLANNING

The OCHL job description, written by the director of the Samuel J. Wood Library (Wood Library) at Weill Cornell Medicine (WCM) and the Oncology Service Line director at NYP, is that of academic faculty librarian. The OCHL reports directly to the assistant director of clinical services at Wood Library; however, the main duties and clinical aspects of the OCHL fall under the oncology department at NYP.

Implementation

The first OCHL joined Wood Library's clinical library services team in December 2017, with plans to develop collateral documentation to promote the new role and oncology information services available to patients/caregivers. The OCHL worked closely with multi-disciplinary teams in the Oncology Service Line and cancer center to disseminate promotional materials and market the new information service and role. Initiatives included developing flyers geared toward both patients/caregivers and providers, attending and presenting at oncology faculty meetings and support groups, participating in oncology committees and workgroups, attending staff huddles and patient experience meetings, and spearheading development of a patient family advisory council (PFAC) specific to the cancer population.

The implementation process involved working collaboratively with the EMR (Epic) team in Information Technology Services (ITS) to develop a built-in referral process for providers to send patients for OCHL services and information therapy appointments. The OCHL attended planning meetings with ITS and hospital administration to discuss, develop, and test the referral process. The OCHL attended four Epic training sessions before being granted access to the system.

Monitoring

Through one-on-one update meetings with cancer center leadership and academic mentors, the OCHL devised a plan to track all patient/caregiver interactions in Epic. The OCHL conducts follow-up with all patients in an effort to ensure information is helpful for discussing and communicating with providers. Documentation of patient encounters in Epic is an important way to report and monitor information interventions between the OCHL and patients/caregivers, and Epic access allows the OCHL to communicate easily with providers about an information therapy appointment or encounter with patients/caregivers. This ensures consistency and transparency for providing information therapy and educational interventions to patients/caregivers. Documenting information therapy paves the way for future data-mining opportunities to research and analyze the impact of information services on patient care, patient empowerment, improvement of patient-provider communication, and influence on overall health outcomes and quality of life.

Evaluating

Discussion defining the methodology for surveying patients/caregivers continues between the Oncology Service Line leadership and the OCHL. Delivery, content, and level of risk—determined by the WCM Institutional Review Board (IRB)—remain to be determined. Anecdotal feedback from providers and patients/caregivers has been positive and well received. Pre- and post-tests measuring effects of the OCHL intervention on patient/caregiver experience include, but are not limited to, assessing the impact of information therapy on patients'/caregivers' understanding of medical conditions, diagnoses and treatment, ease of communicating with providers, improving quality of life, and interest in participating in patient- and family-centered care.

WORKFLOWS AND PARTNERSHIPS FOR LIBRARIANS IN EMRS

The OCHL participates in numerous workgroups, committees, and patient/ caregiver experience meetings. The embedded nature of the OCHL's clinical role fosters partnerships and collaborations on patient-centered care (PCC) initiatives and projects with providers. OCHL assistance improves clinical workflows by providing biomedical literature to clinicians to support innovative treatment methods and goals to develop PCC initiatives. The OCHL annotates meeting minutes, fills information requests from providers, and gathers feedback from patients/caregivers to share with the health care team.

Established Workflow

In partnership with cancer center administrative and clinical leaders, the OCHL embarked on a process for seeing new chemotherapy and/or biotherapy treatment patients/caregivers at two outpatient infusion locations on campus. The clinical workflow for seeing these patients consisted of:

- receiving daily new-patient list;
- reviewing patient's visit history, primary diagnosis, and provider's assessment plan in the EMR;
- compiling consumer/patient material on diagnosis, treatment, nutritional coping concerns, and effective communication with medical team (materials depend on patient case determined through chart review);
- visiting infusion site at time of patient appointment;
- checking in with charge nurse to determine location of patient;
- checking in with patient's individual nurse or nursing team to discuss unique patient concerns;
- reviewing materials with patient/caregiver (if present);
- asking if there are any unanswered questions or information needs;
- leaving contact information with patient/caregiver;
- escalating any clinical concerns of patient/caregiver to nursing staff;
- documenting patient encounter in EMR through chart note template;
- sending follow-up message to patient through patient portal (or phone call if preferred); and
- recording patient follow-up to other members of the patient's care team to document information therapy.

See figure 5.1 for an example of this workflow.

Librarian Initiates EMR Contact

The described workflow for visiting patients/caregivers at cancer infusion locations was tested and succeeded on a technical level but was not as productive as hoped. Meeting patients/caregivers during infusion treatments was beneficial as an introduction to the OCHL role and services available; how-

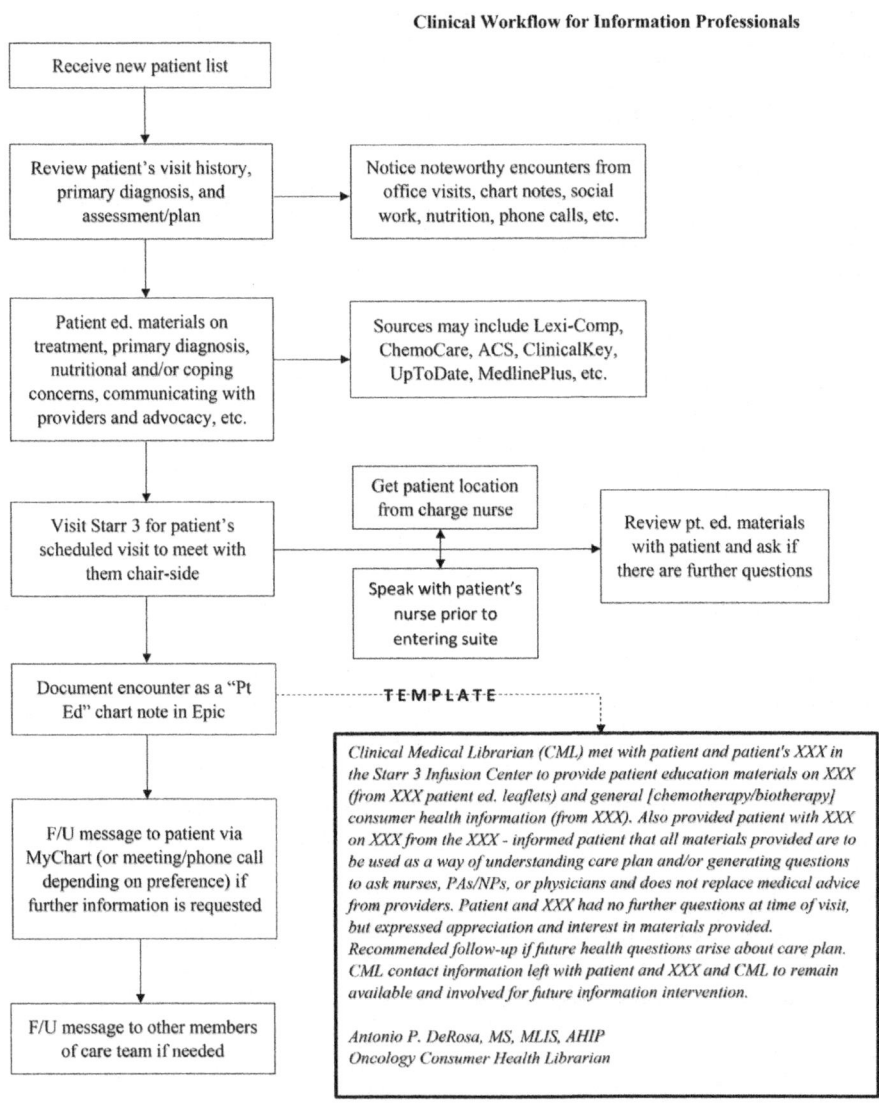

Figure 5.1. Example of Workflow for Clinical Librarians Seeing Patients

ever, it did not address patient/caregiver questions at their most needy time. Patients/caregivers usually have the most questions about their medical care and health immediately following a diagnosis.[8] The OCHL noticed that patients who were already receiving infusion treatment had few questions about their care plan or treatment decisions.

Although the OCHL continues to visit patients at infusion suites, the creation of an updated workflow for meeting patients/caregivers at their most critical point of information need is much more satisfying for everyone. Recognizing newly diagnosed patients have higher needs for information, the OCHL reaches out to patients/caregivers before treatment begins. The OCHL initiates communication via the patient portal of the EMR. The introductory message includes a brief introduction to the OCHL role as well as quick tips for evaluating health and medical information on the internet. This introductory method increased interaction with patients/caregivers and raised the number of information therapy requests and sessions. Patients/caregivers introduced to OCHL services early in the process of treatment decisions have more time to digest information and raise new questions.

Practice Automates EMR Contact

The OCHL collaborated with providers of a specific oncology practice location to pilot an automated information therapy intervention. This practice referred all new patients to the OCHL using the capabilities of Epic established by the Information Technology Service. The referral process is seamless and similar to initiating referrals to other allied health professionals such as social workers, financial councilors, or nutritionists, and so on. Practice providers choose "Cancer Librarian" from a list of available referring services in Epic. The patient/caregiver whose referrals are placed into the OCHL's queue are contacted to schedule an information therapy appointment. This workflow proactively targets patients/caregivers at the outset of their cancer diagnosis. While this referral workflow is still in the pilot phase, the results are very promising.

The automation of referrals in the EMR has led to an increase in the number of patient interactions and encounters. This is an effective way of communicating with patients and delivering introductory information on the role of the OCHL as well as quick tips on searching for health and medical information online. The OCHL enjoys a more streamlined process of receiving patient referrals, connecting with patients to inquire about information needs, and scheduling information therapy counseling sessions to further deliver information and demonstrate consumer health and other medical resources.

HEALTH SEMINARS

The OCHL sponsors and coordinates health education seminars on a variety of topics led by oncologists and other allied health professionals. The seminars are marketed to the public, and this sponsorship promotes the OCHL program, provides exposure for information services available to patients/caregivers, and allows clinicians to engage with patients/caregivers in a non-clinical setting. Discussions during and after the seminars occur often and benefit both patient/caregiver and provider.

PATIENT AND FAMILY ADVISORY COUNCIL (PFAC)

Engaging in a Patient and Family Advisory Council (PFAC) is a vital role for the OCHL. PFACs are intended to be driven by patients for the benefit of patients, families, and caregivers.[9] The PFAC consists of a group of patients/caregivers (advisors) and hospital/college staff (liaisons) working together to improve patient satisfaction and outcomes. Discussions include patient/caregiver experiences and provide critical feedback on clinic and patient areas and practices. The OCHL serves as a liaison member and recruits advisors to join the council. Involved in a wide variety of clinical meetings and hospital committees, the OCHL enjoys a unique opportunity to facilitate goals and recommended actions of the PFAC by creating connections and networks between the advisors and other clinical providers.

PREDICTING FUTURE DIRECTIONS

Embedding information specialists into clinical settings is not a new service model; however, a new paradigm for providing information specialists with EMR charting access for direct patient care encounters is only now gaining increased support.[10] Clinical librarians at other institutions are increasingly gaining access to EMRs to document their activity.

Barriers to offering next-level information services to patients/caregivers exist. Leadership buy-in is essential, and institution-wide outreach and presentation of the benefits of information therapy must be continued. Clinical providers must be made aware of the information needs of their patients and the benefit of leveraging clinical librarians' skills to meet those needs. PFACs provide tremendous information for administrators and clinical providers; the success of PFACs depends on providers encouraging patients/caregivers to participate in the process. There is great opportunity for clinical medical librarians to become increasingly involved in their institutions' PCC initiatives by joining or encouraging the development of PFACS.

More research and evaluation in the area of clinical information services and information therapy for patients/caregivers is needed. Specifically, the profession would benefit from quantitative and data-driven analyses of services offered and measured outcomes.

NOTES

1. Centers for Medicare and Medicaid Services, "Defining Clinicians," www.cms.gov/Medicare/Quality-Initiatives-Patient-Assessment-Instruments/MMS/QMY-Clinicians.html; National Institutes of Health, "NCI Dictionary of Cancer Terms," *National Cancer Institute*, www.cancer.gov/publications/dictionaries/cancer-terms/def/clinician.

2. R. M. Epstein, K. Fiscella, C. S. Lesser, and K. C. Stange, "Why the Nation Needs a Policy Push on Patient-Centered Health Care," *Health Aff* (Project Hope) 29, no. 8 (2010): 1489–95. doi:10.1377/hlthaff.2009.0888.

3. D. W. Kemper and M. Mettler, "Information Therapy: Prescribing the Right Information to the Right Person at the Right Time," *Manag Care Q* 10, no. 4 (2002): 43–46; M. Mettler and D. W. Kemper, "Information Therapy: Health Education One Person at a Time," *Health Promot Prac* 4, no. 3 (2003): 214–17. doi:10.1177/1524839903004003004.

4. Dr. David M. Nanus, Mark W. Pasmantier Professor of Hematology and Oncology in Medicine and chief of the division of hematology and medical oncology at Weill Cornell Medicine.

5. M. McMullan, "Patients Using the Internet to Obtain Health Information: How This Affects the Patient-Health Professional Relationship," *Patient Educ and Counsel* 63, no. 1–2 (2006): 24–28. doi:10.1016/j.pec.2005.10.006; J. Kivits, "Informed Patients and the Internet: A Mediated Context for Consultations with Health Professionals," *J Health Psychol* 11, no. 2 (2006): 269–82. doi:10.1177/1359105306061186; J. McCormack and G. Elwyn, "Shared Decision Is the Only Outcome That Matters When It Comes to Evaluating Evidence-Based Practice," *BMJ Evidence-Based Med* 23, no. 4 (2018): 137–39. doi:10.1136/bmjebm-2018-110922.

6. N. D. Berkman, T. C. Davis, and L. McCormack, "Health Literacy: What Is It?" *J Health Commun* 15, Suppl 2 (2010): 9–19. doi:10.1080/10810730.2010.499985; N. D. Berkman et al., "Low Health Literacy and Health Outcomes: An Updated Systematic Review," *Ann Internl Med* 155, no. 2 (2011): 97–107. doi:10.7326/0003-4819-155-2-201107190-00005.

7. K. J. McCaffery et al., "Addressing Health Literacy in Patient Decision Aids," *BMC Med Inform Decis Making* 13, Suppl 2 (November 2013): S10. doi:10.1186/1472-6947-13-S2-S10.

8. D. L. Roter, "Patient Participation in the Patient-Provider Interaction: The Effects of Patient Question Asking on the Quality of Interaction, Satisfaction and Compliance," *Health Education Monographs* 5, no. 4 (1977): 281–315. doi:10.1177/109019817700500402; A. Dimoska et al., "Can a 'Prompt List' Empower Cancer Patients to Ask Relevant Questions?" *Cancer* 113, no. 2 (2008): 225–37. doi:10.1002/cncr.23543; T. J. Judson, A. S. Detsky, and M. J. Press, "Encouraging Patients to Ask Questions: How to Overcome 'White-Coat Silence,'" *JAMA* 309, no. 22 (2013): 2325–26. doi:10.1001/jama.2013.5797.

9. S. M. Locatelli et al., "Provider Perspectives on and Experiences with Engagement of Patients and Families in Implementing Patient-Centered Care," *Healthcare* (Amsterdam, Netherlands) 3, no. 4 (2015): 209–14. doi:10.1016/j.hjdsi.2015.04.005; A. E. Sharma et al., "'How Can We Talk about Patient-Centered Care without Patients at the Table?' Lessons Learned from Patient Advisory Councils," *J Am Board Fam Med* 12;29, no. 6 (2016): 775–84.

10. S. A. Fowler et al., "Electronic Health Record: Integrating Evidence-Based Information at the Point of Clinical Decision Making," *JMLA* 102, no. 1 (2014): 52–55. doi:10.3163/1536-5050.102.1.010; M. Teixeira, D. A. Cook, B. S. E. Heale, and G. Del Fiol, "Optimization of Infobutton Design and Implementation: A Systematic Review," *J Biom Inform* 74 (October 2017): 10–19. doi:10.1016/j.jbi.2017.08.010.

Chapter Six

Practicing Public Health

Timothy Roberts

DEFINING THE ROLE

"The prime objective or purpose of a public health [librarian] is to collect and make readily accessible all basic knowledge necessary for the prevention of disease and the promotion of health." Swapping out the word *librarian* for *library*, that is a direct quote from Flora Herman's 1956 description of the purpose of public health libraries.[1] The medium and tools used to gather and share knowledge are radically different from those used in 1956, but the purpose of promoting health knowledge remains the same. In this chapter I provide an overview of duties, employment opportunities, preferred resources, some best practices, and services usually provided by public health librarians, although selecting which aspects public health librarianship to highlight for review is similar to the inherent difficulties of herding cats.

Public health librarian Kris Alpi argues that health sciences librarians "are all public health."[2] This view is easy to accept considering the primary responsibility of medical librarians—informing, educating, and empowering patients and providers about health issues[3]—is so closely aligned with one of ten essential public health services listed by the Centers for Disease Control and Prevention (CDC), "to inform, educate, and empower people about health issues."[4]

It is important to understand definitions of key intertwining concepts in the field before delving further into how librarians support public health research. A high-level definition for public health is what "we as a society do collectively to assure the conditions in which people can be healthy."[5] At its core, public health practice promotes healthy behavior in a community and protects the community from injury or disease through policies, health education, and direct patient outreach and research. Public health includes every-

63

thing from aging to zoonosis, and domains include epidemiology, biostatistics, infectious disease control, social and behavioral determinates of health, health policies and systems, environmental and occupational health, community health education, and global health.

The modern practice of public health began in England during the mid-nineteenth century, when John Snow convinced physicians and the public of the relationship between contaminated water at the Broad Street Pump and an outbreak of cholera.[6] *Population health* is a newly emerging dimension of public health that provides "an opportunity for health care systems, agencies and organizations to work together in order to improve the health outcomes of the *communities* they serve."[7] Population health includes health outcomes and patterns of health determinants; researchers focus on the intersectionality of multiple determinants and the links between policies and interventions.[8]

Public health informatics (PHI), the "systematic application of information, computer science and technology to public health practice, research and learning,"[9] includes designing, implementing, and evaluating systems in practice and research, thereby facilitating communication, surveillance, information, and education.[10] Although closely aligned with information technology infrastructure, PHI concentrates on the *way* data is cataloged to enable rapid identification and use of data *rather than how* the technology is written or constructed.[11] Public health practitioners use informatics in daily work duties, increasing and sharing the health knowledge base.[12] Public health informatics includes *population health informatics*, *global health informatics*, and other aspects of *population health*.

The need for expert information systems allowing quick interchanges of knowledge and data is increasingly important as researchers seek to address the intersectionality of public health disciplines, the social determinants of health, and population interventions. Appreciating the complexity of PHI is crucial for librarians to understand. It challenges them to break from seeking information solely from traditional venues. See figure 6.1 to view the relationship between areas of health informatics.

FINDING A JOB

Public Health Librarian in an Academic Medical Center Library

Academic medical centers are familiar settings for librarians specializing in public health. Value-based health care, a plan in which payments to hospitals and physicians are tied to health outcomes of patients, is a typical model for academic medical centers.[13] Social determinants of care become more important when institutions' bottom lines are on the line. For example, a hospital that provides the best cancer treatment available fails if patients leaving the hospital lack social resources to support health outcomes. Opportunities

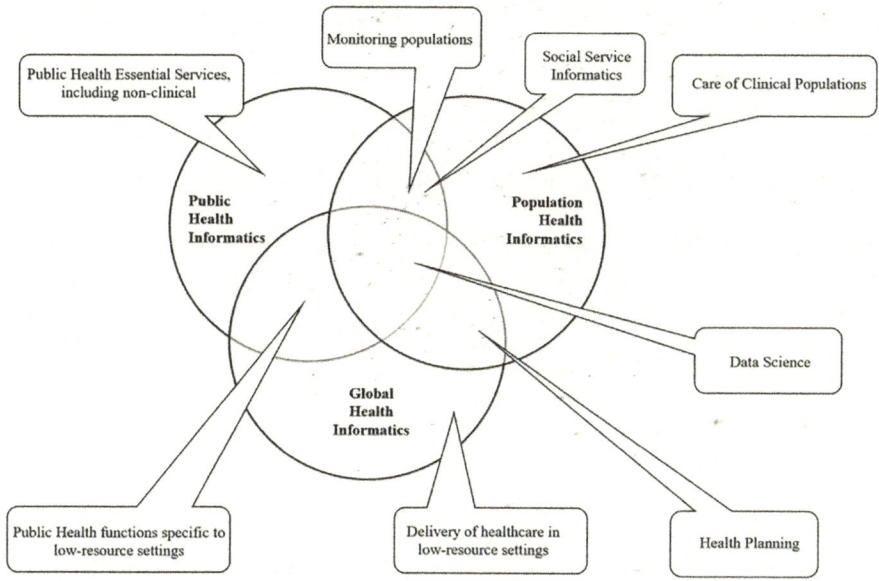

Figure 6.1. Relationship between Areas of Informatics. *Based on J. Lamy et al.,* *"Toward a Formalization of the Process to Select IMIA Yearbook Best Papers,"* **Methods of Information in Medicine 54, no. 2 (2015)**

for librarians exist at academic medical centers that devote valuable resources to interdisciplinary teams researching ways to reduce inequities and disparities caused by negative social determinants of health. Two highly sought-after skills at which librarians usually excel—networking and building interdisciplinary partnerships—were identified in a needs assessment for public health researchers conducted by health librarians at the University of Minnesota.[14]

A public health librarian at an academic medical center usually liaises with members of the Department of Public/Population Health and collaborates on systematic or other literature reviews; instructs new faculty, staff, and medical students in information-management skills; oversees collection development; and curates guides to public health resources.

Academic Public Health Librarian

Undergraduate and graduate institutions not affiliated with medical schools also offer degrees or training in public health and related disciplines. Similar to the academic medical center environment, librarians consult with students, provide research assistance, and teach information and resource use. Because information literacy skills are so important for undergraduates, librarians' responsibilities may be more closely aligned with the course curriculum than at academic medical centers.[15] Some librarians teach semester-long courses in evidence gathering, research methods, and resources.[16] As courses in PHI increase in the curriculum of graduate and undergraduate Public Health education,[17] librarians expand their role to focus on data topics.

Public Health Librarian in the Public Health Agency

Many state public health agencies still maintain a library with a selection of print and electronic materials and employ a librarian to serve needs of both staff and members of the public. There has, however, been a trend toward eliminating this position in agencies and establishing collaboration with academic librarians to fill in the gaps.[18]

Do I Need an MPH?

The need for a second master's degree is actively debated in most fields of librarianship.[19] There are advantages to obtaining a master's in public health (MPH). At a very minimum, the MPH provides you with the vocabulary of the field and a deeper understanding of ways in which the knowledge you are providing will be enacted into policies and interventions. Core to any MPH programs are courses in biostatistics and epidemiology. Having a deeper understanding in these fields is universally applicable when searching and appraising the health-care literature. The research methods curricula in an MPH program—both quantitative and qualitative—serve the practice of medical librarianship well.

IDENTIFYING IMPORTANT RESOURCES

Journals

Given the broad territory covered by public health research, there is no one *best* public health journal. The Science Citation Index (SCI) from Clarivate Analytics Public, Environmental & Occupational Health category is based on a limited definition of *public health*. A better option might be to review a survey conducted by the U.S. Centers for Disease Control and Prevention (CDC) to determine the most highly valued journals used by their researchers.[20] Results from this survey are a valuable resource for selecting journals. See figure 6.2 for titles most used by researchers at the CDC. Members of MLA's Public Health/Health Administration Section (PH/HA) are curating a core list of public health journals that is manageable but also captures the breadth of the field. PH/HA members may access the in-progress version of the list.

Databases

Public health is a broad field. The literature spans many subject areas and comes in a variety of formats, including standard journal articles, governmental and nongovernmental reports, websites, pamphlets, and so on.[21] In addition to biomedical databases such as PubMed and Embase, public health librarians must branch out to include other resources in searches:

- Public Health Partners (PHP; https://phpartners.org/ph_public)—developed in 1997 and maintained by a collaboration of U.S. government agencies, public health organizations, and health sciences libraries—is an important resource for the public health workforce. PHP provides timely, convenient access to selected public health resources on the internet, literature, reports and guidelines, and funding information.[22]
- GIDEON, a web-based global infectious disease management tool, is a key resource for students and researchers interested in global health. GIDEON's diagnosis tool, information on diseases and organisms, and bioterrorism stimulator are used to educate students and clinicians on signs and symptoms associated with bioterrorism agents. GIDEON is an up-to-date and comprehensive resource for geographic medicine.[23]

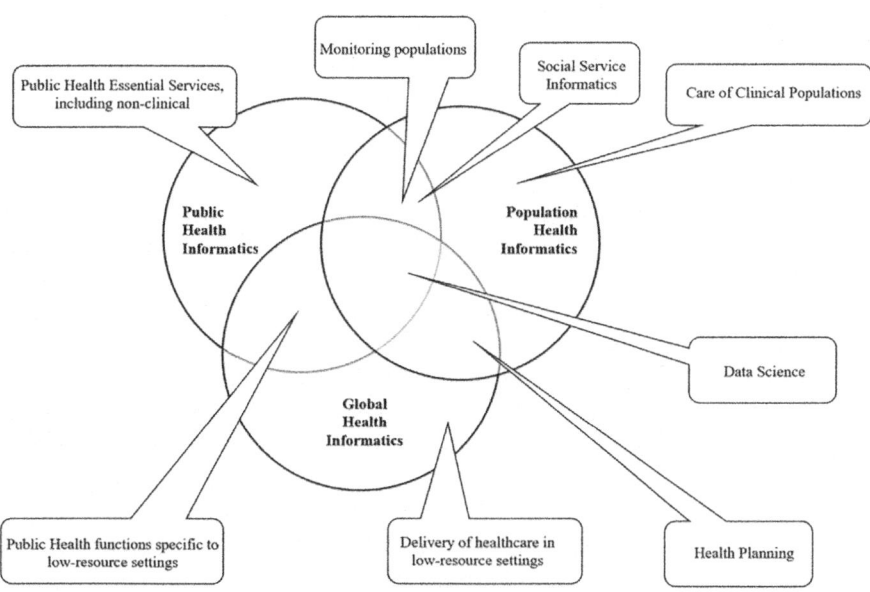

Figure 6.2. Most Downloaded and Most Published Journals by CDC Epidemiologists

- Global Health, produced by CAB International, indexes publications on communicable tropical and parasitic diseases, human nutrition, community and public health, and medicinal and poisonous plants. Coverage begins in 1920 and provides a significant number of unique citations not indexed in MEDLINE.[24]
- ABI/INFORM and Nexis Uni are two business databases that index and abstract articles from business and management publications, dissertations, working papers, regulatory standards, and legal rulings. These citations may inform research about community health campaigns or other health marketing research.[25]
- Ageline, an EBSCO database, focuses on issues of aging and topics relating to people over the age of fifty. Ageline provides perspective from fields of sociology, social work, health sciences, psychology, economics, and public policy. Information format includes book chapters, reports, dissertations, consumer guides, and educational videos.[26]
- GenderWatch and LGBT Life. When conducting research on topics related to underrepresented groups, it is important to explore literature from the group's voice. GenderWatch covers issues on gender and women's studies and lesbian, gay, bisexual, and transgender (LGBT) research.[27] LGBT Life, an EBSO database, indexes core LGBT studies journals, monographs, and other publications.[28]

SYSTEMATIC REVIEW DATABASES

The methodology of conducting systematic literature reviews for public health questions differs slightly from that of clinical questions. Best practices for public health systematic reviews are located in the *Guide to Community Preventive Services: Systematic Reviews and Evidence-Based Recommendations*.[29] These include forming interdisciplinary teams, carefully selecting interventions, and *most importantly*, assessing the quality of evidence. When assessing the quality of evidence, researchers have found that tools that evaluate studies following a public health framework, like the *Effective Public Health Practice Project Quality Assessment Tool*, can provide different determinations than the clinical gold standard *Cochrane Risk of Bias Tool*.[30] Specific tools have been developed to accommodate other study designs,[31] even non-randomized studies.[32] Librarians can play a key role in a systematic review team by identifying the right risk-of-bias tool and overseeing its use.

Regardless of topic, searches for biomedical systematic reviews should combine Embase, PubMed/MEDLINE, Web of Science (Core Collection), and Google Scholar. For certain topics, specialty databases such as CINAHL (Nursing) and PsycINFO (Psychology/Psychiatry) should be included.[33] Those databases are a good start for a public health systematic review, but there are more to consider, and each research project will have a different answer regarding which and how many databases. The search must be reproduced across multiple interfaces, so consider that from the outset and plan accordingly. There are strategies that can improve your efficiency when moving from database to database.[34]

GRAPPLING WITH BIG DATA

It is increasingly important for health data to be discoverable, accessible, and understandable as data sharing and reproducibility become a requirement of the research process.[35] There is no field where data is more important than public health. Most public health data qualifies as "Big Data."[36] Big Data in health care has great variety, high velocity and is often reused making it difficult to extract meaningful information.[37] Big or small, data is pointless if it cannot be understood and communicated; new and inventive ways to visualize Big Data must continue to be developed.[38]

Public health librarians are responding to the call. Librarians, many self-taught, are developing expertise in this area and offering patrons assistance through consultations, formal classes, and drop-in clinics.[39] In 2011, the Association of Research Libraries E-Science Institute produced the "building blocks" of a strategic agenda for e-research.[40] Five years later, NLM's new director, Patti Brennan, positioned NLM to become the hub of data science at NIH. Brennan envisioned NLM as a platform for biomedical discovery and data-powered health. Often researchers are not aware of what librarians bring to the table. It is important that librarians model their description, discovery, and organization skills when interacting with public health research teams.

The ability to easily discover data sets is highly valued. Librarians at New York University Health Sciences Library developed a data catalog after interviewing their researchers about collecting, managing, storing, and preserving their data. A clear need for organizing and identifying data sets emerged from the interviews.[41] "Cataloging" datasets clearly fell in the librarians' wheel house. Based on initial work at NYU, the Data Catalog Collaboration Project (DCCP; www.datacatalogcollaborationproject.org) was created to facilitate the discovery of biomedical research data that are hard to find. The DCCP's goal is to increase the visibility of institutional biomedical research data and encourage other researchers to make use of the data. The collaboration grew to include eight academic health centers in its first few years of existence. Data catalogs from consortium members are currently found through Google Dataset search (https://toolbox.google.com/datasetsearch).

Good clinical research data management starts with a data management plan that describes how data will be collected and managed during the life of a research project. The best management plans include processes for preserving and making data accessible after the project is completed. A good plan requires many of the organizing, cataloging, and archiving skills that librarians have. Consulting with researchers as they develop data management plans and teaching formal classes in best practices is a goal for public health librarians. Fortunately there is a good deal of knowledge sharing within the library community.[42]

As data sharing expands and new research is being done with existing data sets, the ideal is to standardize collection methods and terminology. NLM is the central coordinating body for clinical terminology standards. Searching through NLM's repository of data sets may reveal data standards from previous projects that could be applied to current research. Best practices include this search strategy. A very powerful method librarians can employ when helping researchers design their data sets is to find examples of other projects that are similar enough to use as a model for their research for data standards. Librarians have the ability to find other studies to identify best practices and to catalog repositories of like instruments.[43]

Many libraries now offer researchers courses on data management practices. These efforts have often been collaborations between data-savvy librarians and research specialists. Offerings have included Fundamentals of Data Management, Program using R, Building a Database in RedCap, Data Visualization Tools and Best Practices, Legal Considerations around Data Sharing, and Using Data-Mapping Programs.[44] Librarians looking for a good place to start can seek out established curricula that have been evaluated and refined like the Teaching Toolkit developed by the New York University Health Sciences Library through a grant from the NIH Big Data to Knowledge initiative.[45]

CONCLUSION AND PLACES TO GO FOR MORE INFORMATION

Medical Library Association and the Public Health/Health Administration (PH/HA) Section

First and foremost, join the Medical Library Association and the Public Health/Health Administration (PH/HA) Section. The section operates around the core principle that the fields of public health and health administration are there to communicate relevant health information; account for health-care priorities, policy, and delivery; manage crises; and address major health concerns. As these activities are information intensive and vital places for the exchange of ideas and best practices, PH/HA programs not only demonstrate the importance of public health informatics but also point to its growing significance on an international and global scale.

Along with the list of core journals mentioned previously, section members can apply for an award through the Sewell Memorial Fund, which provides funding for librarians to attend the American Public Health Association Annual Meeting. Attending the meeting with a cohort of librarians to share experiences and reflections can be a great way to expand your understanding and skills in public health librarianship. A requirement of the award is to have a mentor in the field of public health and spend time participating at a booth or moderator. Both help you integrate into the conference and the field.

American Public Health Association

Even if you do not apply for the Sewell award, consider joining the American Public Health Association (APHA) or your state local chapter. Attending APHA conferences and seeing the research being done is the best way for you to connect your skills and interests and think of ways you can contribute to the field.

NOTES

1. F. E. Herman, "Symposium on Types of Medical Libraries. VIII. The Public Health Library," *Bull Med Libr Assoc* 43, no. 2 (1955).

2. K. M. Alpi, "We Are All Public Health," *J Med Libr Assoc: JMLA* 95, no. 3 (2007).

3. M. A. Banks, K. W. Cogdill, C. R. Selden, and M. A. Cahn, "Complementary Competencies: Public Health and Health Sciences Librarianship," *J Med Libr Assoc: JMLA* 93, no. 3 (2005).

4. Centers for Disease Control, "Public Health System & the 10 Essential Public Health Services," www.cdc.gov/publichealthgateway/publichealthservices/essentialhealthservices.html.

5. Institute of Medicine, *The Future of Public Health* (Washington, D.C.: National Academy Press; 1988).

6. J. P. Vandenbroucke, H. M. Eelkman Rooda, and H. Beukers, "Who Made John Snow a Hero?" *Am J Epidemol* 133, no. 10 (1991).

7. Centers for Disease Control, "What Is Population Health?" www.cdc.gov/pophealthtraining/whatis.html.

8. D. Kindig and G. Stoddart, "What Is Population Health?" *Am J Pub Health* 93, no. 3 (2003).

9. W. A. Yasnoff, P. W. O'Carroll, D. Koo, R. W. Linkins, and E. M. Kilbourne, "Public Health Informatics: Improving and Transforming Public Health in the Information Age," *J Pub Health Manag Pract* 6, no. 6 (2000).

10. B. L. Massoudi and K. G. Chester, "Public Health, Population Health, and Epidemiology Informatics: Recent Research and Trends in the United States," *Yearbook Med Informatics* 26, no. 1 (2017).

11. T. G. Savel and S. Foldy, "The Role of Public Health Informatics in Enhancing Public Health Surveillance," *MMWR* Supp 61, no. 3 (2012).

12. F. Williams, A. Oke, and I. Zachary, "Public Health Delivery in the Information Age: The Role of Informatics and Technology," *Perspect Public Health* (2019).

13. Anonymous, "What Is Value-Based Healthcare?" *NEJM Catylst* (2017). Published electronically January 1, 2017, https://catalyst.nejm.org/what-is-value-based-healthcare.

14. S. L. Hunt and C. J. Bakker, "A Qualitative Analysis of the Information Science Needs of Public Health Researchers in an Academic Setting," *J Med Libr Assoc: JMLA* 106, no. 2 (2018).

15. L. Cobus, "Integrating Information Literacy into the Education of Public Health Professionals: Roles for Librarians and the Library," *J Med Libr Assoc: JMLA* 96, no. 1 (2008).

16. M. L. Le, "Information Needs of Public Health Students," *Health Info Libr J* 31, no. 4 (2014).

17. X. Yu et al., "Developing an Evidence-Based Public Health Informatics Course," *J Med Libr Assoc:JMLA* 103, no. 4 (2015); K. Gray, "Public Health Platforms: An Emerging Informatics Approach to Health Professional Learning and Development," *J Pub Health Res* 5, no. 1 (2016).

18. J. Barr-Walker, "Evidence-Based Information Needs of Public Health Workers: A Systematized Review," *J Med Libr Assoc:JMLA* 105, no. 1 (2017).

19. J. Ferguson, "Additional Degree Required? Advanced Subject Knowledge and Academic Librarianship," *portal: Libraries and the Academy* 16, no. 4 (2016).

20. J. Iskander et al., "Articles Published and Downloaded by Public Health Scientists: Analysis of Data From the CDC Public Health Library, 2011-2013," *J Public Health Manag Pract* 22, no. 4 (2016).

21. E. Aalai, C. Gleghorn, A. Webb, and S. W. Glover, "Accessing Public Health Information: A Preliminary Comparison of CABI's GLOBAL HEALTH Database and MEDLINE," *Health Info Libr J* 26, no. 1 (2009).

22. M. A. Cahn et al., "The Partners in Information Access for the Public Health Workforce: A Collaboration to Improve and Protect the Public's Health, 1995-2006," *J Med Libr Assoc: JMLA* 95, no. 3 (2007).

23. S. A. Berger, "GIDEON: A Comprehensive Web-Based Resource for Geographic Medicine," *Int J Health Geogr* 22, no. 4 (2005).

24. Aalai, Gleghorn, Webb, and Glover, "Accessing Public Health Information."

25. L. M. Schwartz and S. Woloshin, "Medical Marketing in the United States, 1997-2016," *JAMA* 32, no. 1 (2019).

26. E. Vardell and B. M. Linares, "AgeLine: A Database of Social Gerontoloy Literature," *Med Ref Serv Q* 32, no. 3 (2013).

27. C. Ingold, "Women's Studies Databases: A Critical Comparison of Three Databases for Core Journals in Women and Gender Studies," *Library Trends* 56, no. 2 (2007).

28. K. Antell, "The Citation Landscape of Scholarly Literature in LGBT Studies: A Snapshot for Subject Librarians," *Coll Res Libr* 73, no. 6 (2012).

29. P. A. Briss et al., "Developing an Evidence-Based Guide to Community Preventive Services—Methods," *Am J Prev Med* 18, no. 1 (2000).

30. S. Armijo-Olivo et al., "Assessment of Study Quality for Systematic Reviews: A Comparison of the Cochrane Collaboration Risk of Bias Tool and the Effective Public Health Practice Project Quality Assessment Tool: Methodological Research," *J Eval Clin Pract* 18, no. 1 (2012).

31. M. J. Page, J. E. McKenzie, and J. P. T. Higgins, "Tools for Assessing Risk of Reporting Biases in Studies and Syntheses of Studies: A Systematic Review," *BMJ open* 8, no. 3 (2018): e019703.

32. J. A. Sterne et al., "ROBINS-I: A Tool for Assessing Risk of Bias in Non-Randomised Studies of Interventions," *BMJ* 355 (2016): i4919.

33. W. M. Bramer, M. L. Rethlefsen, J. Kleijnen, and O. H. Franco, "Optimal Database Combinations for Literature Searches in Systematic Reviews: A Prospective Exploratory Study," *Syst Rev* 6, no. 1 (2017).

34. W. M. Bramer, G. B. de Jonge, M. L. Rethlefsen, F. Mast, and J. Kleijnen, "A Systematic Approach to Searching: An Efficient and Complete Method to Develop Literature Searches," *J Med Libr Assoc:JMLA* 106, no. 4 (2018).

35. A. Surkis and K. Read, "Research Data Management," *J Med Libr Assoc:JMLA* 103, no. 3 (2015).

36. O. Ola and K. Sedig, "The Challenge of Big Data in Public Health: An Opportunity for Visual Analytics," *Online Journal of Public Health Informatics* 5, no. 3 (2014): 223.

37. Ola and Sedig, "The Challenge of Big Data in Public Health."

38. L. N. Carroll et al., "Visualization for Big Health Data," *Online J Public Health Inform* 5, no. 3 (2014).

39. M. D. Brandenburg and R. Garcia-Milian, "Interinstitutional Collaboration for End-User Bioinformatics Training: Cytoscape as a Case Study," *J Med Libr Assoc:JMLA* 105, no. 2 (2017); F. W. Z. LaPolla and D. Rubin, "The 'Data Visualization Clinic': A Library-Led Critique Workshop for Data Visualization," *J Med Libr Assoc:JMLA* 106, no. 4 (2018); Carroll et al., "Visualization for Big Health Data"; O. Ola and K. Sedig, "Beyond Simple Charts: Design of Visualizations for Big Health Data," *Online J Public Health Inform* 8, no. 3 (2016); M. M. Catalano, P. Vaughn, and J. Been, "Using Maps to Promote Data-Driven Decision-Making: One Library's Experience in Data Visualization Instruction," *Med Ref Serv Q* 36, no. 4 (2017).

40. Association of Research Libraries, "Overview of the ARL/DLF E-Science Institute," www.arl.org/focus-areas/telecommunications-policies/1087-overview-of-the-arldlf-e-science-institute-.XH7SdFNKiys.

41. K. B. Read et al., "Starting the Data Conversation: Informing Data Services at an Academic Health Sciences Library," *J Med Libr Assoc:JMLA* 103, no. 3 (2015).

42. K. B. Read, "Adapting Data Management Education to Support Clinical Research Projects in an Academic Medical Center," *J Med Libr Assoc:JMLA* 107, no. 1 (2019); T. P. Bardyn, E. F. Patridge, M. T. Moore, and J. J. Koh, "Health Sciences Libraries Advancing Collaborative Clinical Research Data Management in Universities," *J Escience Librariansh* 7, no. 2 (2018).

43. Read, "Adapting Data Management Education."

44. Brandenburg and Garcia-Milian, "Interinstitutional Collaboration for End-User Bioinformatics Training"; A. Surkis, F. W. LaPolla, N. Contaxis, and K. B. Read, "Data Day to Day: Building a Community of Expertise to Address Data Skills Gaps in an Academic Medical Center," *J Med Libr Assoc:JMLA* 105, no. 2 (2017); S. Zhao, "A New Training Program: Biomedical and Health Research Data Management for Librarians," Blog, *Teaching Resources & Tips Guide*, https://news.nnlm.gov/nto/2017/09/20/a-new-training-program-biomedical-and-health-research-data-management-for-librarians.

45. K. R. Read, C. Larson, C. Gillespie, So Young Oh, and A. Surkis, "Teaching Toolkit," PLOS One (accepted for publication).

Chapter Seven

Presenting Clinical Resources in Novel Ways

Antonio P. DeRosa, Michelle Demetres, Keith C. Mages, Loretta Merlo, Peter Robert Oxley, Judy C. Stribling, Michael Wood, Drew Wright, and Terrie R. Wheeler

OVERVIEW (ANTONIO P. DeROSA)

In a time of the twenty-four-hour news cycle pumping information at lightning speed and the increasing pressure on academic faculty to avidly pursue and disseminate their research, it can be difficult for even the most information-savvy person to keep up on breaking events and new discoveries. This is especially true in the medical profession where new treatments, techniques, and findings are reported every day. In addition to navigating the realm of published medical literature, clinicians are expected to practice evidence-based medicine to deliver the best possible care to their patients. Clinicians need to know how to access and navigate clinical resources if they expect to deliver exceptional patient care, but staying current in the dynamic landscape of their field is a daunting task for physicians, residents, fellows, medical students, and other clinical staff. Enter the clinical medical librarian (CML).

By curating key clinical resources and educating clinicians on tools to support their decision-making practices, CMLs offer a unique set of skills to raise awareness and promote the importance of choosing the right resource at the right time to make the best evidence-based decisions when caring for their patients. Socrates said, "True knowledge exists in knowing that you know nothing." CMLs work with clinicians to bridge the gap between their medical knowledge and the bourgeoning research and evidence in their fields.

To address the need for accessible and easy access to clinical resources, librarians at Weill Cornell Medicine (WCM) have developed programs, activities, and presentations to assist both established and future clinicians. For those in the learning stages of their careers, including medical students and residents, WCM librarians have developed focused LibGuides for the anesthesiology residency program and evidence-based medicine targeting first-year medical students. Engaging "Spinning the Wheel" exercises presented during neurology clerkship instructional sessions helps third-year medical students learn how to pose effective clinical questions and search the literature. The librarians run an annual treasure hunt designed to introduce incoming medical students to the robust resources and services offered by the Samuel J. Wood Library (Wood Library) at WCM. Clinical staff and other faculty can take advantage of weekly Tech Tuesday Talks aimed at demystifying technology and providing guidance on using technology services to enhance clinical practice (e.g., using Jupyter notebooks to manage data-intensive projects). Also, the annual SMARTFest event held in the Wood Library brings together the medical college and affiliate hospital communities for resource demonstrations, access to vendors, and information about the services and resources available to support their clinical needs. This chapter will detail each of these programs and resources from the perspective of the WCM librarians involved in their development and ongoing success.

CURATED LIBGUIDES

Anesthesiology (Michael A. Wood)

In 2014, the New York–Presbyterian/Weill Cornell Medicine's Anesthesiology Department established a digital curriculum for its residency program. One of the objectives was to eliminate the need for printed textbooks for their residents and provide electronic access to textbooks and other resources via iPads. The department reached out to the library's assistant director for clinical services and head of resource management for assistance in establishing a portal to access the library's content via the iPads.

Prior to launch of the digital curriculum, the department spent significant funds to acquire several printed textbook titles for each resident throughout their residency. See table 7.1 to compare title and cost differences in 2008 and 2019.[1] In 2008, at least eight anesthesiology textbooks were already available in electronic format and accessible by residents and students on and off campus.

The library coordinated with the department's director of education and chief resident to curate a list of resources including e-books, e-journals, and mobile apps for the program. Springshare's LibGuide platform was ideal for creating the portal. The library pays an annual cost for the vendor-hosted

Table 7.1.   Anesthesiology Resources in 2008 and 2019

2008	2019
https://web.archive.org/web/ 20080907191255/http:// www.nycornell.org/anesthesiology/ residency/benefits.html	https://anesthesiology.weill.cornell.edu/ education/residency-program/benefits- and-salary

Memberships and Book Allowances
We encourage our residents to build their own professional library, first by giving them "the basic" textbook, and later by giving them a book allowance of $300.00 to purchase texts in areas of special interest.

Memberships, Resources, and Academic Allowances
We encourage our residents to begin building their own professional library. In addition to the textbooks, educational resources, and academic allowances listed below, all fees associated with the Basic and Advanced examinations of the ABA are fully reimbursed.

PGY-2 CA-1 ($300 Book Allowance)
- NYSSA/ASA Membership (includes a subscription to the journal *Anesthesiology*)
- IARS Membership (includes a subscription to the journal *Anesthesia & Analgesia*)
- Miller & Stoelting's *Basic of Anesthesia*
- Miller's *Anesthesia* (2 volumes + 2 CDs)
- Hemming's *Foundations of Anesthesia*
- Brown's *Atlas of Regional Anesthesia*

Interns ($200 Book Allowance)
- iPad with remote all to all e-books, e-journals, and apps held by the Weill Cornell Medical Library.
- Barash's *Clinical Anesthesia Fundamentals*, 1st ed.
- Hemming's *Pharmacology and Physiology for Anesthesia: Foundations and Clinical Application*, 1st ed.
- Yao and Artusio's *Anesthesiology: Problem-Oriented Patient Management*, 8th ed.

CA-1 Year ($300 Book Allowance)

PGY-3 CA-2 ($500 Book Allowance)
- Jaffe's *An Anesthesiologist's Manual of Surgical Procedures*

CA-2 Year ($500 Book Allowance)

PGY-4 CA-3 ($700 Book Allowance)
- Allowance can be used toward board exams
- Stoetling's *Anesthesia and Co-Existing Diseases*
- Benumoff's *Anesthesia and Perioperative Complications*
Rathmell's *Regional Anesthesia: The Requisites in Anesthesiology*

CA-3 Year ($700 Book Allowance)

LibGuide. The department LibGuide is publicly accessible here: http:// med.cornell.libguides.com/c.php?g=761656.

A great benefit of utilizing the LibGuide platform and many of the library's other electronic resources is that they are mobile friendly, mobile optimized, or developed with responsive design to facilitate access on iPads, tablets, and mobile phones.

Anesthesiology residents' iPads and iPhones were pre-configured with a shortcut to the curated LibGuide and access to the Wi-Fi networks of both the college and the hospital. This facilitated seamless and transparent access to the resources. Additionally, off-campus access was made possible through EZproxy and VPN client.

The residents can access hundreds of e-books and e-journals from clinical resources such as Elsevier's Clinicalkey and Wolters Kluwer's Books@Ovid as well as web and app versions of ClinicalKey, DynaMed, UpToDate, and Visual Dx.

As reported on the college's website on January 13, 2017, "The Department of Anesthesiology Residency Program at Weill Cornell Medicine and NewYork-Presbyterian has been recognized as an Apple Distinguished Program for its success in creating a digital learning environment using mobile technology." It further stated, "The Apple Distinguished Program designation is reserved for programs that meet criteria for innovation, leadership and educational excellence, and demonstrate a clear vision of exemplary learning environments."[2]

Evidence-Based Medicine (Michelle Demetres, Keith C. Mages)

As part of the first-year medical curriculum, the WCM library faculty participates in a health, illness, and disease "How to Find an Answer," evidence-based medicine (EBM) session. This two-hour session is one of a series of EBM classes developed collaboratively with WCM physicians and designed to introduce students to the EBM process. Harvesting the simple technology of LibGuides, WCM librarians curated important learning materials and seamlessly integrated them into the medical student curriculum.

This class begins with physician faculty introducing the following clinical scenario to the student group:

> You are seeing a sixty-five-year-old woman with hypertension, hyperlipidemia, type 2 diabetes mellitus, and chronic kidney disease (stage 3). You notice that the patient's LDL cholesterol is elevated to 140 (normal is less than 70 to 100). The patient is not taking statin. You counsel the patient about statin use. She states she does worry about having a heart attack since her brother had one recently, but a friend told her statins do not work in patients with kidney disease. Additionally, she is worried about developing myopathy. You want to research literature to review effectiveness of statin therapy for a patient like yours.

Students are asked to construct a clinical question using the PICO(T) framework. Next, a faculty librarian introduces the library-constructed EBM subject guide to the group. Using the LibGuide as a roadmap, students take a deeper dive into the EBM process. Charts and graphs illustrate the steps of EBM. The librarian begins by introducing "The 5 A's": Assess, Ask, Acquire, Appraise, and Apply. Discussion then moves on to question types (therapy, diagnosis, prognosis, etiology/harm, prevention, clinical exam, and cost) and the most appropriate studies used to address each of these particular questions. All steps are adapted from JAMAevidence's *Users' Guides to Medical Literature* (third edition).[3] Haynes's *Integrated "5S" Levels of Organization of Evidence Pyramid*, depicting the levels of evidence and appropriate EBM resources available to students, is also highlighted.[4]

The group is briefly introduced to PubMed and its search mechanics. The introduction includes an overview of MeSH, Booleans operators, truncation, phrase searching, filters and sorting, and clinical queries.

The final hour of the class is dedicated to small-group breakout sessions. Faculty librarians guide groups of approximately fifteen medical students through the initial clinical scenario. The PICO(T) for this scenario is reiterated, appropriate databases/resources are discussed, and students are required to locate quality literature addressing the topic at hand. Students are encouraged to use the LibGuide, in particular an EBM worksheet guided by the principles of the five A's as a resource. This worksheet asks students to answer the following questions and considerations:

1. What is your scenario?
2. What type of question are you asking?
3. What are your background questions? List names of sources consulted.
4. What is your PICO?
5. Clearly and concisely state your foreground question.
6. What study type is best suited for answering this type of question?
7. What resource(s) did you choose to search in?
8. Delineate your search strategy in writing.
9. List the articles you will choose to appraise.
10. To what extent are the results valid?
11. Present your recommendations as if you are talking to your "patient."

If time allows, students review the following additional clinical scenario:

You are seeing a fifty-five-year-old healthy man in office for a well visit. You recommend screening colonoscopy. The patient reports that nobody in his immediate family has history of colon cancer and questions the benefits of

colon cancer screening. You decide to search for studies evaluating effectiveness of colonoscopy in decreasing mortality from colon cancer.

It is important to mention students are not required to use one resource
over another (e.g., PubMed); they are encouraged to use what will best answer the clinical question. After students complete the worksheet, a volunteer
student from each groups presents their findings in an open discussion environment. Librarians promote dialogue of the issues encountered and the pros
and cons of resources to introduce strengths and peculiarities of different
databases.

TREASURE HUNT (DREW WRIGHT, LORETTA MERLO)

Much has been written about the Millennial generation—the tech-savvy,
team-oriented, selfie-snapping, optimistic high-achievers born between 1982
and 1996. In 2006, many of this generation began entering graduate school.

With the characteristics of Millennials in mind, the staff of Wood Library
at WCM set out to create an engaging orientation for the medical school's
freshman class. Library-sponsored scavenger hunts have been successfully
implemented at several institutions and show positive results regarding student engagement.[5] The Library Treasure Hunt at WCM, now in its thirteenth
year, was designed as a team activity, appealing to the students' competitive
natures, incorporating technology, and most importantly, beginning their education in how to find and use reliable medical information online in the age
of Wikipedia and Google.

The format of the treasure hunt has remained constant: students are given
a map of the physical space and a clue—in limerick format—that challenges
each team to find a different station inside the library. At each station, staff
members tell the students about a library service, resource, or policy; have
them complete a task; and then provide them with the next clue. This allows
students to become familiar with the physical layout of the library, meet
library staff, and use some medical resources before classes even begin. For
example, at a station meant to introduce electronic resources, students are
shown how to navigate the library's webpage to access and demo a clinical
point of care tool.

As technology has evolved, so has the treasure hunt—instead of paper
clues in envelopes, students now access each clue by scanning a QR code
using their tablets. One clue requires them to post team photos with their best
"pirate face" on the library's Facebook page. They take a final quiz on their
tablets (this *is* medical school, after all) and use our chat service, which
provides a date and time stamp, to signal their team's completion of the hunt.
The team with the fastest time and the highest score on the quiz wins.

As technology continues to change, the methodology and tools will have to be updated. For example, fewer and fewer incoming medical students use the same social media platforms that previous classes have used. This has required the library to remain informed on popular digital trends and adjust the clues and tasks accordingly. Due to the success of the treasure hunt, other departments (including the university archives and information technology) on campus have expressed interest in participating in future iterations.

In addition to training incoming medical students, the treasure hunt also serves as the library's first opportunity to solicit feedback from them. A satisfaction/assessment survey was built to develop a baseline of skill sets, potential avenues of interest in future skills, and preferred learning styles, in addition to gathering feedback on the treasure hunt experience itself.[6]

SPINNING THE WHEEL: NEUROLOGY CLERKSHIP (JUDY C. STRIBLING)

Third-year students on the in-patient portion of their neurology clerkship at WCM are required to attend two library-led sessions to refresh their searching and acquiring information skills; eleven rotations of neurology clerkships are offered each academic year. The goals of these sessions are to review EBM concepts and PICO question formation, highlight Wood Library resources, and reinforce the importance of lifelong learning. Upon completion of the library sessions, clerkship students formulate a clinical question based on a patient seen during the clerkship and search, acquire, analyze, and apply the results. Students have a two-week window to complete the assignment and fill out a worksheet housed in Canvas—WCM's Course Management System—containing their search strategy, most applicable clinical study category for the question, analysis of the content of results, and applicability to patient.

The first thirty-minute session consists of a review of the library website and special subject guides created to support EBM and neurology. Instructions for completing a five-point quiz and EBM worksheet are located in Canvas. The second library session focuses on searching different resources to answer clinical neurology questions and takes place in the library's computer lab classroom. The CML observed that students were distracted by having access to computers and spent a great deal of their class time working on other assignments, using instant messaging, or catching up on e-mail rather than focusing on search strategies and biomedical resources.

To address this, the CML changed the seminar location. And, realizing the importance of exposing students to resources other than UpToDate or Google Scholar, understanding the competitive nature of medical students, and creating enthusiasm and fun in the learning environment, the CML instructor devised a competitive game approach to engage students' interest and participation in the learning process.

Now, instead of taking place in a computer lab, the search session is held in a regular conference room with one computer connected to a wall-mounted monitor. Following a general discussion of EBM, using the PICO formula to create good clinical questions and choosing appropriate resources to answer questions, students volunteer to "Spin the Wheel."

The wheel—an old-fashioned fortune wheel—panels contain a clinical question or some other query related to biomedical research databases. (See figure 7.1 to view a representation of the wheel.) The CML asks a volunteer to start the process by spinning the wheel and searching for the answer to the question on the landing panel. If no one rises to the occasion, the CML reminds students that each panel could represent a patient in their current practice. This gentle cajoling generally moves the most competitive student to volunteer to take a spin.

Questions and clinical scenarios included on the wheel are based on actual clinical experiences of previous neurology clerkship students or on important aspects of using popular biomedical databases and are purposefully non-intimidating. The CML and other students may suggest search strategies to the volunteer during his or her turn at the wheel. Usually the volunteer searches at least two different databases to find an answer. The CML offers critique of the different resources and may suggest consulting a resource rarely used by students. After the first volunteer, other students generally become increasingly eager to take a turn at the wheel.

At the conclusion of the wheel search session, the CML asks students if they learned anything new during the session. Anecdotally, the author reports students enjoy the playful nature of the exercise and express appreciation for the CML's time and expertise. Since initiating the wheel, more students make research appointments and communicate more frequently with the CML.

SMARTFEST (TERRIE R. WHEELER)

Two years ago, a faculty survey revealed that WCM faculty wanted access to several tools that were already available to them, indicating a need to increase awareness of library resources. How best to achieve this? Human beings often learn best when they are having fun. While WCM CMLs put increased effort into engaging new faculty and introducing them to the suite of resources available to them, we also developed an annual technology fair called SMARTFest. Wood Library holds this annual event in February after the holidays and before spring break, right when the community needs a distraction from the winter weather. While this started as a humble division

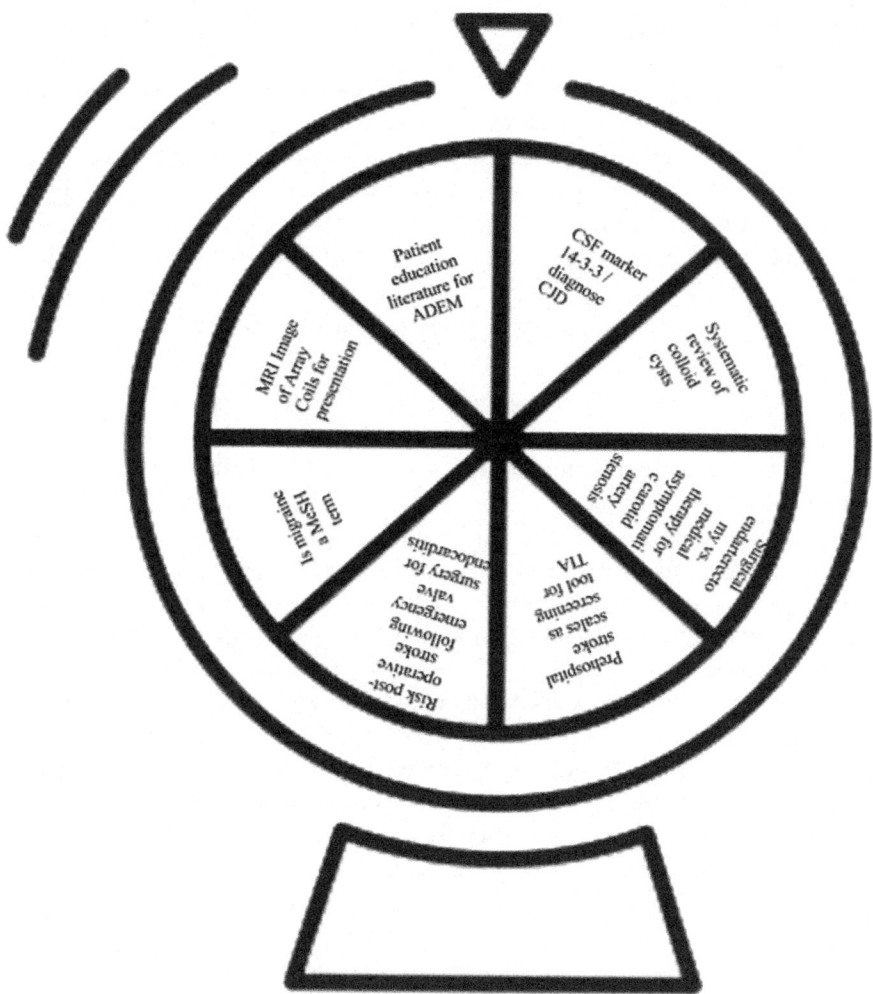

Figure 7.1. Spin the Wheel

event, it has grown into a college-wide celebration that engages users of all types: administrators, academic faculty, residents, nurses, and students. There is something for everyone at SMARTFest.

And as a medical school, there are a lot of clinical resources to demonstrate. Vendors of clinical resources pay to attend the event, giving them firsthand interaction with users of their products. The vendors are able to show users best practices for interacting with their products; the practices vary based on the user's needs or use case. Feedback from the vendors each year is very positive. They report that downloads and usage of their product peaks at WCM during these annual fairs, and users continue to engage with their products afterward. This past February WCM CMLs instituted our first "user feedback" live survey, and users reported how much they learned about the resources available to them. This user feedback told us a lot about why SMARTFest resonates with our community.

Each year we evaluate our successes and failures to see what we can do the following year to make the event bigger and better. SMARTFest allows us to introduce clinical resources to our users in an engaging way while they learn and have fun. See table 7.2 for five years of SMARTFest statistics.

TECH TUESDAY (PETER ROBERT OXLEY)

To help clinicians (and all community members) navigate the increasing number of electronic applications now required for clinical practice and re-search, a weekly open seminar was started in the library for medical, re-search, and administrative staff and students. The goal of these "Tech Tues-days" is to help users become familiar with how to access and use electronic resources provided through Information Technology Services. Tech Tuesday seminars are presented by internal experts or staff with extensive experience using the tools. The format is typically a half-hour, in-person presentation, held in the library common space. No pre-registration is required, but partici-pants sign in to track attendance and enable delivery of electronic resources.

Applications or tools that are part of an extensive software suite (e.g., Adobe or Microsoft Office) are presented as part of special monthly series and advertised in the lead-up to the series. Slides and other electronic re-sources are delivered to the participants following the seminar.

Topics cover a broad range of applications and services, from software suites (Adobe, Microsoft Office), storage services (Box, Secure Read Archive), computation (Amazon Web Services), technology (Microsoft Sur-face Hub, 3D printing), and clinical research services (i2b2, Architecture Research Computing in Health [ARCH], Data Core, REDCap), to research applications (Jupyter notebooks, Qualtrics, Endnote, myNCBI).

Table 7.2. Five Years of SMARTFest Statistics

SMARTFest Statistics	2015	2016	2017	2018	2019
# of Vendors	7	16	18	21	25
Sponsor Donations	<$2K	$13.5K	$14.8K	$15.5K	$25.4K
# WCM Booths	16	21	25	26	30
# of Visitors	610	1,118	1,030	1,150	1,587

Since the kickoff of Tech Tuesdays in April 2015, WCM has hosted 153 sessions with 2,545 participants. While average attendance is seventeen participants, some consistently popular sessions such as an introductory Microsoft Excel seminar, can draw as many as eighty participants. See figure 7.2 for the top ten classes offered at Tech Tuesday. Five of the top ten most-attended sessions covered a feature of Microsoft Excel; three of the top ten presented Adobe software; the remaining two top ten sessions were about Endnote and i2b2. Attendance at Tech Tuesday events continues to grow, from an initial attendance of 449 in 2015 to 844 participants in 2018.

Jupyter Notebooks: A Typical Tech Tuesday, Introduction (Peter Robert Oxley)

In an era of evidence-based practice, translational science, and precision medicine, it is becoming ever more important to enable clinicians to be able to access and interact with the data underlying their clinical decisions. Yet due to the disparate publication and storage of each of these elements, links between data, analysis, results, and interpretation can be vague and difficult to identify. This is a problem not only for interpretation but also for reprodu-

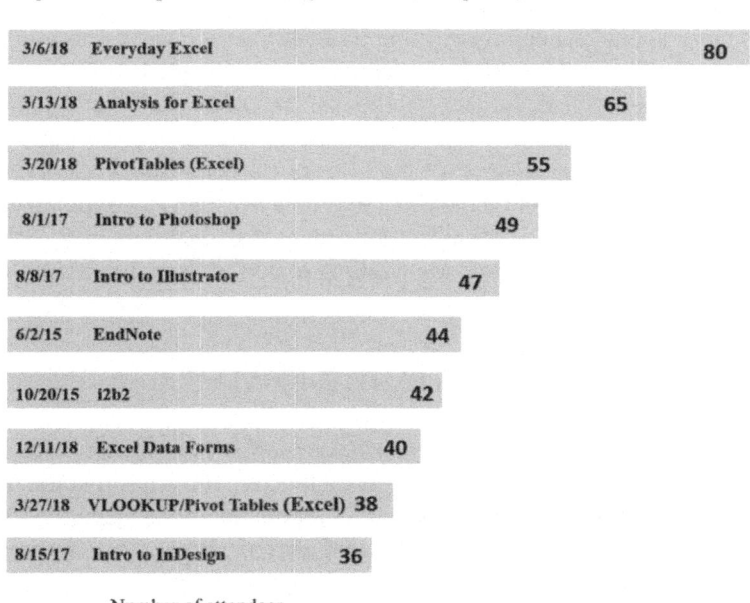

Top Ten Most Popular Tech Tuesday Sessions since April 30, 2015

Date	Session	Attendees
3/6/18	Everyday Excel	80
3/13/18	Analysis for Excel	65
3/20/18	PivotTables (Excel)	55
8/1/17	Intro to Photoshop	49
8/8/17	Intro to Illustrator	47
6/2/15	EndNote	44
10/20/15	i2b2	42
12/11/18	Excel Data Forms	40
3/27/18	VLOOKUP/Pivot Tables (Excel)	38
8/15/17	Intro to InDesign	36

Number of attendees

Figure 7.2. Top 10 Tech Tuesday Talks

cibility, findability, and accessibility. Jupyter notebooks are one of the more recent attempts to address this problem, and use of the notebooks is experiencing rapid growth and garnering support from a number of large corporate players.

In brief, Jupyter electronic notebooks allow the integration of formatted, narrative text, executable code, and analytical output (both tabular and graphical) into a single, linear, interactive document. Jupyter notebooks can be shared with stakeholders for re-execution or alteration of the underlying algorithms, or in static form, to allow understanding of the relationships between a research question, methodology, analysis, results, and interpretation. Jupyter is an open-source project, developed by a large and diverse community, making it available to institutions with meager resources. Notebooks can also be hosted for free by platforms such as MyBinder.org and dryad.org, or uploaded into repositories such as github. They can support over a dozen languages, including the commonly utilized statistical languages SPSS, SAS, and MATLAB.

At the Wood library, the bioinformatics service includes the provision of basic analytical services, combined with consultation to help clinician-researchers understand the analysis, so they can correctly interpret them. In order to facilitate this goal, WCM runs analyses in Jupyter notebooks, as a means of both performing and sharing the work with our patrons. WCM librarians also run regular workshops on how to use Jupyter, and the most commonly used languages within this environment (Python and R).

As grant agencies begin specifying more stringent data-research-management plans, all members of the research team will need to become more facile with tools such as Jupyter notebooks. As collaborators and supporters of the research enterprise, libraries similarly need to become equipped to utilize these tools. The creation of the Library Carpentry data science curriculum by the Carpentries organization, and its corresponding rapid growth in courses run and attended, bears testament to the fact that many libraries already recognize this fact, and are working to add to their informatics expertise.

CONCLUSION (ANTONIO P. DeROSA)

Showcasing resources and library services to support clinical practice can be done in innovative and entertaining ways. Gone are the days of static links to key books and websites and lists of bibliographic databases peppering library websites. The discovery of new technologies has allowed for dynamic and interactive research guide development like the content-focused anesthesiology and EBM guides presented in this chapter, as well as robust programs like Jupyter to manage and analyze complex datasets. Nontraditional avenues of delivering instruction like Tech Tuesdays and novel instructional methods like Spinning the Wheel have engaged clinical learners in new ways. Even out-of-the box ideas for promoting clinical resources and services like SMARTFest and the treasure hunt are good ways to raise awareness and draw attention to what the library and librarians have to offer in support of clinical needs. CMLs have the ability to position themselves precisely in view of clinicians and clinicians-in-training to act as a pipeline to the resources needed by these users to succeed in practice. And they can have fun while doing it.

NOTES

1. Department of Anesthesiology, "Residency Program," Weill Medical College of Cornell University and New York–Presbyterian Hospital, https://web.archive.org/web/20080907191255/www.nycornell.org/anesthesiology/residency/benefits.html; Weill Cornell Medicine, "Benefits and Salary," Anesthesiology, https://anesthesiology.weill.cornell.edu/education/residency-program/benefits-and-salary.

2. "Anesthesiology Residency Program Named an Apple Distinguished Program," Weill Cornell Medicine, Office of External Affairs, https://news.weill.cornell.edu/news/2017/01/anesthesiology-residency-program-named-an-apple-distinguished-program.

3. G. Guyatt, R. Drummond, M. Meade, and D. Cook, *Users' Guides to the Medical Literature: A Manual for Evidence-Based Clinical Practice*, 3rd ed., vol. 706 (New York: Mcgraw-Hill Education, 2015).

4. R. B. Haynes, "Of Studies, Syntheses, Synopses, Summaries, and Systems: The '5s' Evolution of Information Services for Evidence-Based Healthcare Decisions," [In eng] *Evid Based Med* 11, no. 6 (December 2006): 162–64.

5. S. Marcus and S. Beck, "A Library Adventure: Comparing a Treasure Hunt with a Traditional Freshman Orientation Tour," *College & Research Libraries* 64, no. 1 (2003): 23–44; K. Thompson, L. Knapp, and R. Kardos, "From Tourist to Treasure Hunter: A Self-Guided Orientation Programme for First-Year Students," *Health Information and Libraries Journal* (2008); S. Stormes, "Butler Freshmen Hunt for Library Treasure," *Librarian Scholarship* (1993): 7.

6. J. Richardson, D. Bouquin, L. Tmanova, and D. Wright, "Information and Informatics Literacies of First-Year Medical Students," [In eng]. *J Med Libr Assoc* 103, no. 4 (October 2015): 198–202.

Chapter Eight

Journey to Magnet

*A Nursing-Librarian Collaboration for
Nursing Excellence*

Marisol Hernandez

This chapter provides a brief description of the Magnet Recognition Program (MRP) and describes how a clinical librarian (CL) embedded in the nursing department at a major cancer center collaborated with administrators and nursing staff on the Magnet journey. Throughout this chapter, the word *Magnet* refers to the certification program and denotes status, certification, recognition, and other factors associated with the program.

In the late twentieth century, a convergence of poor working conditions and negative perceptions of the career led to a nursing shortage crisis in the United States. In 1983, the American Academy of Nursing (AAN) responded by assigning a Task Force on Nursing Practice in Hospitals to explore how some hospitals succeeded in retaining nurses during the shortage. In 1990, the American Nurses Credential Center (ANCC) incorporated as a subsidiary of the AAN to provide credentialing services to hospitals. Evolution of initial task force work resulted in today's MRP, which is designed to help hospitals recruit and retain qualified nurses and to recognize those that are successful in doing so.[1] Achieving "Magnet" status requires strategic and budgetary commitment from hospital leadership and organization-wide dedication to the goal. Earning Magnet status is a significant accomplishment, representing thousands of dollars of investment and many hours of hard work.

The "Journey to Magnet" is lengthy, expensive, and not linear. On average, hospitals spend four years and five months to complete Magnet certification, at an annual cost of $500,000, resulting in overall investment of $2.1 million. Researchers calculate hospitals begin to realize payback from achieving Magnet status in two to three years.[2] Awarded for a four-year period, continued Magnet status requires hospitals to reapply for Magnet accreditation, and re-application costs rise annually. Given the significant commitment required to apply, attain, and maintain Magnet status, is it worth the cost? Numerous studies reveal that benefits of Magnet status contribute not only to the hospital's reputation but also to improved patient care and satisfaction.[3] Magnet hospitals have a higher percentage of satisfied nurses and lower nurse turnover and vacancy, both of which improve a hospital's bottom line.

THE NURSING SHORTAGE

Various articles, reports, and papers chronicle the severity of the United States' nursing shortage crisis. Kimball and O'Neil examined the topic in the context of national and global economics and social history. The authors cite the principal causes of the shortage as: the failure of nursing practice to adopt the advancements in medical technology following World War II; the success of the Women's Rights Movement in creating opportunities for women in careers not traditionally viewed appropriate for women; and the irony that the extensive changing financial and administrative requirements occurring in health care could not be addressed by a "profession that lacks the authority to create change within the healthcare system."[4] Evans acknowledges these societal factors but places primary blame for the nursing shortage on negative hospital working conditions, specifically referring to "lack of opportunity for suitable career advancement, burnout, lack of opportunity for professional development, poor nurse-physician relations and lack of recognition by peers and hospital administration."[5]

THE GOLD STANDARD

How were some hospital nursing programs able to retain nurses despite the forces creating the shortage crisis? AAN's task force identified hospital nursing programs with successful practices and outcomes that they labeled Magnet or "Gold Standard Hospitals."[6] Common approaches at these institutions were identified and described as the fourteen Forces of Magnetism (FOM).[7]

- Force 1: Quality of Nursing Leadership
- Force 2: Organizational Structure
- Force 3: Management Style
- Force 4: Personnel Policies and Programs
- Force 5: Professional Models of Care
- Force 6: Quality of Care

- Force 7: Quality Improvement
- Force 8: Consultation and Resources
- Force 9: Autonomy
- Force 10: Community and the Health Care Organization
- Force 11: Nurses as Teachers
- Force 12: Image of Nursing
- Force 13: Interdisciplinary Relationships
- Force 14: Professional Development

In 2008, the MRP developed a new model that grouped the FOMs into six key components: Transformational Leadership, Structural Empowerment, Exemplary Professional Practice, New Knowledge, Innovations and Improvements, and Empirical Quality Results.[8] Hospitals applying for Magnet status recognition from the MRP must demonstrate expertise in the Model and FOMs aligned within the components. See table 8.1 to view the relationship of components and FOMs in the most recent Magnet model.[9]

OPPORTUNITIES FOR LIBRARIANS

A white paper published by the Medical Library Association identified shared core objectives of the MRP. The first sentence of the publication reveals the significance of librarian participation in a hospital's journey to Magnet status. "Excellence in nursing care and patient outcomes begins and ends with appropriate, relevant information to guide healthcare decisions."[10] Working together is mutually beneficial for clinical librarians and nurses. For nurses at Magnet applicant hospitals, an ideal librarian partner should have expertise searching biomedical literature databases, delivering information retrieval and analysis, and teaching search skills to clinical learners as well as previous exposure to clinical environments.[11] For librarians, helping an institution attain Magnet status is a prime opportunity to demonstrate a *positive impact on patient outcomes, patient satisfaction, and hospital financial bottom lines*.

One of the most significant collaborations between librarians and nurses resides in the *New Knowledge, Innovations, and Improvements* Magnet model where clinical librarians, traditionally evidence-based practice (EBP) champions in health-care settings, are valuable resources for nurses who must integrate EBP into their program. EBP, "the conscientious, explicit and judicious use of current best *evidence* in making decisions about the care of the individual patient,"[12] is associated with improved effectiveness and cost-efficiency of health-care delivery, better patient outcomes, and higher quality of care.[13] EBP was originally described as a five-step process:

Table 8.1.   Magnet Models and Forces of Magnetism

MODEL COMPONENTS	FORCES OF MAGNETISM
Transformational Leadership	Quality of Nursing Leadership Force #1 Management Style Force #3
Structural Empowerment	Organizational Structure Force #2 Personnel Policies and Programs Force #4 Community and the Health-Care Organization Force #10 Image of Nursing Force #12 Professional Development Force #14
Exemplary Professional Practice	Professional Models of Care Force #5 Consultation and Resources Force #8 Autonomy Force #9 Nurses as Teachers Force #11 Interdisciplinary Relationships Force #13
New Knowledge, Innovations, and Improvements	Quality Improvement Force #7
Empirical Quality	Quality of Care Force #6

1. Ask the clinical question in PICOT format (Patient Population, Intervention, Comparison, Outcome, Time).
2. Search for the best evidence.
3. Critically appraise the evidence.
4. Integrate the evidence with a clinician's expertise and a patient's preferences and values.
5. Evaluate the outcome of the practice change.

Melnyk and Fineout-Overholt modified the language and steps of EBP to address the needs and culture of nursing practice:[14]

1. Cultivate a spirit of inquiry within an EBP culture and environment.
2. Ask the burning clinical question in a PICOT format.

3. Search for and collect the most relevant best evidence.
4. Critically appraise the evidence (i.e., rapid critical appraisal, evaluation, synthesis, and recommendations).
5. Integrate the best evidence with one's clinical expertise and patient preferences and values in making a practice decision or change.
6. Evaluate outcomes of practice decision or change based on evidence.
7. Disseminate the outcomes of the EBP decision or change.

VIGNETTES FROM MEMORIAL SLOAN KETTERING'S MAGNET JOURNEY

Memorial Sloan Kettering (MSK), one of forty-seven national cancer institutes designated as comprehensive cancer centers, has 473 inpatient beds in New York City and eight ambulatory clinics throughout Westchester County, Long Island, and New Jersey. MSK's nursing staff of close to four thousand was enthusiastically committed to the Magnet journey and enjoyed unwavering support from top leadership including the chief nursing officer and the president of the institution. Long identified as having a strong and talented nursing workforce, MSK's prestigious MRP status provides additional opportunity for nursing staff to demonstrate excellence and obtain national recognition.

Laying the Foundation

The foundation for attaining Magnet status at MSK was set in 2008 when MSK nursing leadership adopted a professional practice model known as Relationship-Based Care (RBC), "which provides a conceptual framework for nursing. RBC integrated nurses' three key relationships—with patients and caregivers, their colleagues, themselves—to create a healing environment where patients and families are at the center of caring practice."[15]

Establishing a Team

The institution hired a Magnet program director who managed the establishment of strategic teams to execute the Magnet mission. Teams included the Magnet Steering Committee, Magnet masters, Magnet writers, and Magnet champions. Charged with surveying the institutional climate and documenting available resources to undertake the Magnet journey, these teams made outreach to nursing staff and additional stakeholders, including the library. Specifically, these teams requested a clinical librarian to provide library orientation presentations, establish a LibGuide on Magnet-related resources, and review documentation for inclusion of relevant library resources and to strengthen the nursing EBP program.

Utilizing the Library

Professional librarians, rotating student interns, and volunteers staff the library at MSK and provide clinicians with access to the most current clinical information through content management, document delivery, scholarly communication, virtual library services, and reference services. The library team supports numerous MSK initiatives by providing quality resources and services to support professional development, enhance workflow, and improve good clinical decision-making for quality patient care. The Clinical Medical Library (CML) Program at MSK includes research informationists (RIs) who liaise with individual clinical departments in the hospital. Established in 2006, the CML relationship with nursing was already in place when MSK's Magnet journey began.

The team was ahead of the goal. For two years, the RIs, library management, and the nursing department worked in tandem. The library acquired appropriate Magnet resources; the RI attended nursing council meetings and developed partnerships with nurse educators, nurse researchers, clinical nurse specialists, nursing students, and members of nursing leadership. The embedded RI developed a strong nursing-library partnership and carefully assessed how the nursing staff searched for information and identified gaps in their knowledge approach. At MSK, the embedded RI conducted surveys designed to elicit nursing information-seeking needs. Survey results led to development of customized library training available in the nursing environment, the library, and online. The RI participated in several nursing continuing education coursework sessions on campus. These courses provided the RI with a better understanding of nursing care, considerations, and implications in the oncology setting.

The RI participated in the orientation of newly hired nursing staff and provided nursing-specific orientation sessions to the library. Some library orientation sessions included small groups; others were individual meetings arranged by the nurse manager/nurse leader. The RI was a member of the Nursing Practice Council and Nursing Research Council. Membership in these councils provided the RI with information and insight into nursing practice issues and nursing research before proposals were submitted to the Institutional Review Board (IRB) for approval. The RI had opportunity to identify possible challenges in research projects and suggest methodology changes before IRB submission, thereby making the research process more efficient. The RI worked with clinical nurse specialists to help with EBP projects assigned to their nursing students conducting clinical rotations at the hospital. The RI also presented at larger nursing venues, including internal Nursing Grand Rounds, and collaborated with nursing staff on scholarly publications, conference posters, and podium presentations. Below are two example scenarios of nurse-librarian collaboration:

Scenario 1

Nurse manager of the Nurse Residency Program approached the RI with proposal to collaborate on an abstract submission for poster presentation at the Annual Congress of the Oncology Nursing Society. The poster highlighted MSK's Nurse Residency Program (NRP) as a vehicle for promoting evidence-based practice (EBP) and provided survey results of questions answered by program participants.

Scenario 2

A nurse anesthetist asked for assistance from MSK library's systematic review service. Assigned to the project, the RI met with the nurse anesthetist and his team to discuss the objective of the review, helped formulate the PICO question, developed inclusion/exclusion criteria, chose databases and citation management software, discussed options for publications (poster and/or journals) and devised a list of keywords and subject headings to search. This systematic review examined clinical practice guidelines on the use of capnography during procedural sedation in radiology. The review was published in a radiology-focused nursing journal.

Magnet Resources

Providing a robust CML program to support educational and research endeavors of a variety of departments in a large complex cancer organization requires resources. The RI advocates for nursing content and negotiates with library management to include resources that support EBP and scholarly communication. Nursing staff have access to databases, tools, and other library services for EBP and other research activities. In addition to the more familiar databases like PubMed and CINAHL (Cumulative Index of Nursing and Allied Health Literature), MSK nurses also have access to the following EBP resources:

- BMJ Best Practice
- Cochrane Library
- Embase
- Johanna Briggs Evidence-Based Practice Database

The library supports scholarly communication by providing access to citation management tools like EndNote and RefWorks. Training on library resources is available through individual appointment, on an ad hoc basis, and through online registration. Training topics include citation management, database searching, EBP, publishing, and author support. Other tools like

LibGuides encourage use of subscribed library products and provide platforms for training.

The RI engages nursing staff at remote MSK ambulatory clinics through
technology. MSK's robust website contains numerous tools and provides
access and technical support for research. The RI uses video conferencing
platforms like GoToMeeting to support other MSK locations. Support includes teaching library classes, consulting with researchers, and leading journal club discussions. The RI provides reference chat service using a number
of technologies including Library H3lp and delivers search results through
citation management tools. The RI updates staff about new library resources
and makes occasional visits to other locations to participate in nursing-specific events.

Opportunities for nursing-librarian partnerships continue to grow as both
professions participate in the fast-changing health-care environment and as
more health-care organizations undertake the Magnet journey. Developments
in medical and nursing research, patient care, and technology will continue to
be the driving force of these collaborations. Because information-seeking
behaviors vary, continuing to converse with stakeholders and engaging with
nursing staff at all levels is key.

Evidence-Based Practice

In 2016, MSK's nursing department engaged the Helene Fuld Health Trust
National Institute for Evidence-Based Practice in Nursing and Healthcare,
based at the Ohio State University's College of Nursing, to deliver an on-site
evidence-based practice immersion session designed to build and sustain
EBP. One hundred nursing staff and the RI attended the five-day workshop
to learn about Ohio State nursing faculty's EBP methodology. The workshop
provided training to the MSK nursing leadership team and other advanced
nurses to assist with the goal of adopting and implementing the methodology
at MSK. The five-day "Evidence Immersion Program" was the first step of a
fifteen-month journey during which designated groups worked on EBP projects designed to enhance nursing practice and improve patient outcomes.
The groups presented their EBP projects and results at the program's concluding internal EBP summit. MSK continues to host the annual immersion
event in order to reach as many of the nursing staff as possible, and the RI
attends each year.

Nurse Residency Program

Accredited by the American Nurses Credential Center (ANCC), the Nurse
Residency Program (NRP) at MSK provides support for nurses transitioning
from undergraduate studies to professional practice. The one-year program

promotes professional practice, critical thinking, and leadership skills through education and clinical activities. The RI delivers an orientation to evidence-based library resources and services and consults with individuals or small groups to support evidence-based posters required for completion of the program.

Nursing Research Fellowship

The Nursing Research Fellowship Program (NRFP), a one-year program for advanced nurses with interest in conducting research, builds capacity and support for nursing research. The NRFP is competitive, with only a select number of slots. The RI introduces databases and other online tools and provides support for scholarly communication and critical appraisal. Similar to the Nurse Residence Program, librarians consult with nursing fellows throughout the program. The ultimate goal of this program is dissemination of fellows' research through publication or conference presentation.

Through either presentations to different clinical groups around the center or ad hoc consultations, the librarian liaison provides guidance to nurses as they prepare the evidence-based presentations required for maintenance of program Magnet status or professional promotion.

In summary, achieving Magnet recognition is the highest distinction for any health-care facility. Magnet demonstrates excellence in nursing with expectations of improved patient outcomes and quality patient care. The prestigious award allows health-care organizations to promote quality nursing clinical practice, provide the delivery of quality patient care, and establish a mechanism for sharing nursing knowledge and best practices. Additionally, it elevates nursing engagement and autonomy, which fosters a safer space for patients, plays a role in better patient outcomes, and contributes to improvements in nursing satisfaction, thus lowering RN turnover.

Furthermore, the Magnet journey provides numerous opportunities for libraries and librarians to collaborate in the areas of instruction, collection development, and most importantly EBP. As a result, MSK nurses are heavily involved in quality improvement projects and disseminate and contribute significant research results at internal and external venues. The partnership between the nursing department and library services at MSK is evidence of a highly successful model.

NOTES

1. "History of the Magnet Program," American Nurses Credentialing Center, www.nursingworld.org/organizational-programs/magnet/history.

2. M. Blair, "Becoming a Magnet Hospital Can Increase Revenue, Offset Costs of Achieving Magnet Status," Robert Wood Johnson Foundation, www.rwjf.org/en/library/articles-and-news/2014/05/becoming-a-magnet-hospital-can-increase-revenue--offset-costs-of.html.

3. A. Kutney-Lee et al., "Changes in Patient and Nurse Outcomes Associated with Magnet Hospital Recognition," *Med Care* 53, no. 6 (2015); S. H. Park, S. Gass, and D. K. Boyle, "Comparison of Reasons for Nurse Turnover in Magnet and Non-Magnet Hospitals," *Journal of Nursing Administration* 46, no. 5 (2016); K. Drenkard, "Going for the Gold: The Value of Attaining Magnet Recognition," *American Nurse Today* 5, no. 3 (2010).

4. B. Kimball and E. O'Neal, "Health Care's Human Crisis: The American Nursing Shortage," Robert Wood Johnson Foundation, 2002, www.rwjf.org/en/library/articles-and-news/2003/01/health-cares-human-crisis-the-american-nursing-shortage.html.

5. S. A. Evans and R. Carlson, "Nurse-Physician Collaboration: Solving the Nursing Shortage Crisis," *Journal of the American College of Cardiology* 20, no. 7 (1992).

6. M. Kramer and C. E. Schmalenberg, "Best Quality Patient Care: A Historical Perspective on Magnet Hospitals," *Nurs Adm Q* 29, no. 3 (2005).

7. "Forces of Magnetism," American Nurses Credentialing Center, www.nursingworld.org/organizational-programs/magnet/history/forces-of-magnetism.

8. "History of the Magnet Program."

9. "Eligibility Requirements," American Nurses Credential Center, www.nursingworld.org/organizational-programs/magnet/eligibility-requirements.

10. M. Allison and M. Bandy, "Magnet Recognition Program Collaboration Proposal," White Paper, 2015, www.mlanet.org/d/do/424.

11. M. B. Liston, "Librarian Involvement in Magnet Criteria: A Focus on New Knowledge, Innovations, and Improvements," *Journal of Hospital Librarianship* 12, no. 2 (2012).

12. D. L. Sackett, *Evidence-Based Medicine: How to Prace and Teach EBM*, 2nd ed. (New York: Churchill Livingstone, 2000).

13. B. M. Melnyk et al., "Correlates among Cognitive Beliefs, EBP Implementation, Organizational Culture, Cohesion and Job Satisfaction in Evidence-Based Practice Mentors from a Community Hospital System," *Nursing Outlook* 58, no. 6 (2010); B. M. Melnyk et al., "The State of Evidence-Based Practice in US Nurses: Critical Implications for Nurse Leaders and Educators," *Journal of Nursing Administration* 42, no. 9 (2012); G. R. Wallen et al., "Implementing Evidence-Based Practice: Effectiveness of a Structured Multifaceted Mentorship Programme," *Journal of Advanced Nursing* 66, no. 12 (2010).

14. B. M. Melnyk, "The Foundation for Improving Healthcare Quality, Patient Outcomes & Costs with Evidence-Based Practice," in *Implementing the Evidence-Based Practice (EBP) Competencies in Healthcare: A Practical Guide for Improving Quality, Safety, and Outcomes*, ed. Bernadette Mazurek Melnyk, Lynn Gallagher-Ford, and Ellen Fineout-Overholt (Indianapolis: Sigma Theta Tau International Honor Society of Nursing, 2016).

15. J. Stallard, "MSK Celebrates Prestigious Recognition for Nursing Excellence," Memorial Sloan Kettering Cancer Center, www.mskcc.org/blog/msk-celebrates-prestigious-recognition-nursing-excellence; G. Guanci, "How Relationship-Based Care Supports the Magnet Journey," *Nursing Management* 47, no. 1 (2016).

Chapter Nine

Educating Clinical Learners

Medical Librarian Roles and Important Considerations

Rachel Pinotti

The ability to effectively find and utilize information is an essential skill for twenty-first-century clinicians. Indeed, Glasziou and colleagues assert, "The skills needed to find potentially relevant studies quickly and reliably, to separate the wheat from the chaff, and to apply sound research findings to patient care have today become as essential as skills with a stethoscope."[1] The evidence-based medicine (EBM) model (i.e., finding, appraising, and applying information to patient care) was novel and even somewhat controversial[2] when it was proposed in the 1990s. In the intervening quarter century, the core skills of the EBM model have been codified into undergraduate and graduate medical education program requirements and widely adopted in medical school curricula.[3]

As expert searchers and evaluators of information, medical librarians are well suited to design and deliver EBM education to clinical learners at both the undergraduate and graduate medical education levels. Beyond instruction, health science librarians play a variety of roles in EBM education, including curriculum development and resource curation.[4] Drawing on the literature and the author's expertise, this chapter will discuss medical librarians' roles in EBM education and suggest important considerations and new tools for use in educating clinical learners.

LIBRARIAN INVOLVEMENT IN EBM INSTRUCTION

Understanding exactly what it is that you need to know and where and how to look for an answer can feel daunting for clinical learners. While librarians play various roles in EBM education, their role in the *ask* and *acquire* steps of the EBM cycle may be the most well established and the most common. Librarians teach in both the pre-clinical and clinical years of medical school, support EBM learning for residents and fellows, and teach in classrooms and at the point of care using a variety of approaches.[5] Specific challenges learners commonly encounter are described below along with ideas and tools for helping to address these challenges, based on the author's observations and experience.

UNDERSTANDING THE QUESTION

A student on their psychiatry clerkship or a psychiatry intern faced with a patient with dissociative symptoms may be more likely to think, "What causes these symptoms?" than "What is the differential diagnosis for patients presenting with dissociative symptoms?" Similarly, an emergency medicine resident helping a patient with a pulmonary embolism (PE) might ask herself, "Do I need to admit this patient?" rather than, "Among patients with PE, what set of clinical features indicate outpatient treatment is a safe option?"

While the Patient-Intervention-Comparison-Outcome (PICO) model has been demonstrated to be a useful framework,[6] formulating PICO questions can be difficult for clinical learners. Lloyd et al. state, "The ability to ask PICO style questions, search for the literature effectively and interpret the search results is not intuitive and requires training."[7] More generally, background questions may need to be adjusted from the way they are likely to occur to a learner into a searchable question. Thus, helping students learn how to convert natural language questions into well-formulated clinical questions and appropriately categorize their question is among the first tasks of the medical librarian. Drawing on several sources,[8] an algorithmic aid developed for this purpose is shown in figure 9.1.

COMMON STUMBLING BLOCKS IN QUESTION FORMULATION

Given medical students' limited knowledge of the literature, it can be challenging for them to know what is reasonable to expect in terms of study populations and clinical outcomes. In the author's observation, these appear to be two of the most common stumbling blocks in PICO question formulation.

The purpose of constructing a PICO question is to utilize it to identify one or more studies that answer the question and ultimately inform a clinical decision. In order to do this, clinical learners must think about a potential clinical study in which their patient would be eligible to participate. Abstracting out from a specific patient to a reasonable clinical study population can

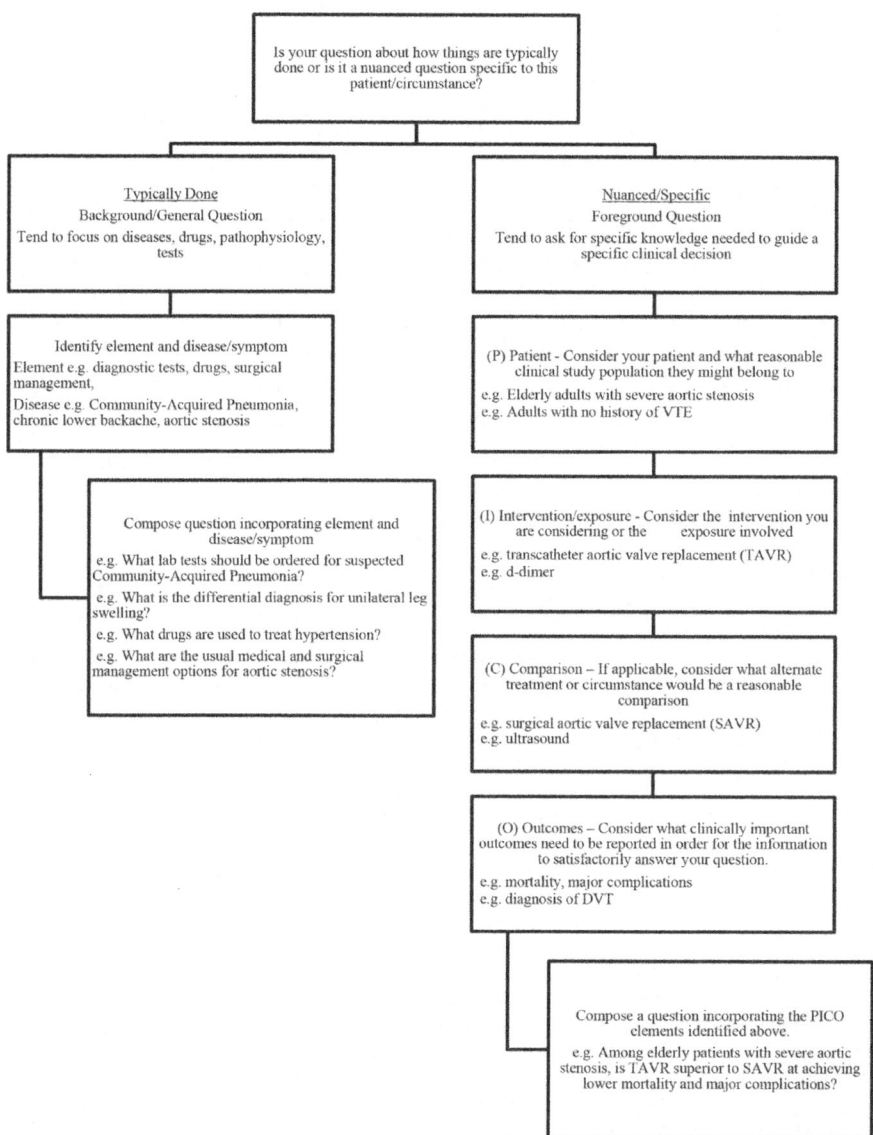

Figure 9.1. Clinical Question Algorithm

be difficult for learners. It requires practice and improves with time and increased familiarity with the medical literature. An example of this process of zooming out from a hypothetical specific patient to a clinical study population that the patient would likely be eligible to participate in is shown in figure 9.2.

Learners face a similar challenge in identifying clinically important outcomes that are reasonable to expect to find when formulating clinical questions. When initially asked to formulate a PICO question, learners tend to list general outcomes rather than identify specific, patient-important outcomes. This may be due to not knowing what outcomes are important for a given condition or due to lack of familiarity with the literature, which limits their ability to know what types of outcomes are typically reported. While an experienced clinician will know that all-cause mortality, stroke, and surgical complications are key outcomes to look for in trials on surgery for aortic stenosis, an early career learner is likely to not yet know this. Similarly, they are often unsure what length of follow-up they can reasonably expect to find in the literature. Would it be reasonable to expect a study to report on key outcomes at thirty days? Ninety days? Two years? An additional challenge with outcomes is the prevalence of surrogate outcomes in the literature. The Biomarkers Definitions Working Group defines a surrogate outcome as "a biomarker that is intended to substitute for a clinical endpoint. A surrogate endpoint is expected to predict clinical benefit (or harm or lack of benefit or harm) based on epidemiologic, therapeutic, pathophysiologic, or other scientific evidence."[9] While surrogate endpoints sometimes accurately predict the clinical benefit they are intended to, this is not always the case. These types of outcomes can be misleading and carry the possibility of diminished benefits and even patient harm.[10]

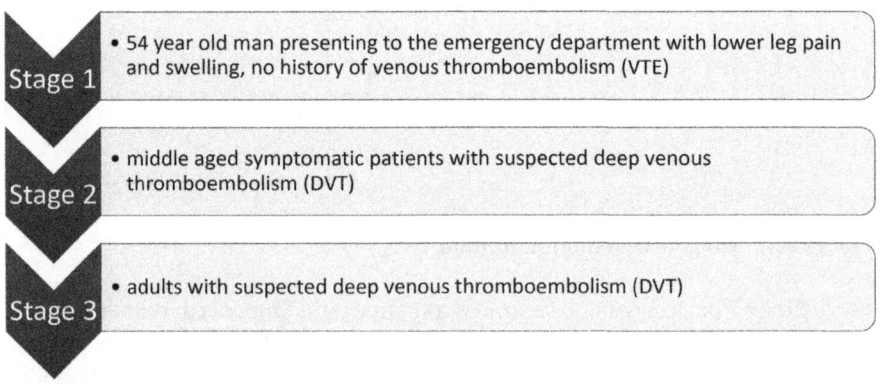

Figure 9.2. From Specific to Searchable

HELPING LEARNERS OVERCOME CHALLENGES IN QUESTION FORMULATION

Maggio and colleagues report that involvement in question formulation instruction is a common role for librarians in EBM education.[11] Identifying the appropriate patient population and outcomes enables learners to acquire the best available evidence to answer their question—studies in which the patient population is a suitable match for their patient in terms of disease state and risk level and that report appropriate, clinically important outcomes. Medical librarians can assist learners in overcoming the difficulties they face in developing and honing these skills in many ways. First and foremost, librarians communicate that developing clinical questions is difficult and takes practice. Students and house staff may be reluctant to admit they find it hard to construct searchable questions, especially in front of their peers. In acknowledging this difficulty, the librarian can earn the status of a trusted advisor, providing support as learners draft and revise their questions.

Research reveals "one-off" instruction sessions may not be sufficient for helping learners attain new skills.[12] Medical librarians have explored different options for integrating education through multiple channels and achieving longitudinal involvement in their institutions' curricula.[13] Multiple, progressive sessions for the same group—whether embedded sessions within the medical school curriculum or didactic sessions for a residency program—will achieve better results. An initial session might begin with a lecture, after which trainees can be given examples of clinical questions and asked to categorize them as either background or foreground and to dissect the PICO elements of the foreground questions. A subsequent session might begin with reviewing the content from the first session, then providing students a clinical vignette and asking them to write their own examples of background and foreground questions. A third session might ask students to generate clinical questions based on their recent clinical experiences. In this way, content is reinforced and students have the opportunity to progressively build up their question-asking skills. Librarians can use these sessions to help learners overcome the difficulties related to selecting the appropriate patient population and outcomes.

SELECTING THE RIGHT RESOURCE TO FIND AN ANSWER

The answers that learners need are heavily dependent on their stage of medical training and the setting in which the question arose. Wyer et al. write that in order for content to be effective, it needs to be modified according to the "teaching venue, period, and competing demands, as well as the learners' previous knowledge, readiness, and inclination to absorb new content."[14]

Despite—or perhaps due to—the plethora of resources and tools available, selecting the right resource to consult given their information need and time constraints can be challenging for clinical learners. Sastre and colleagues have shown that training can improve resource utilization,[15] and Gaines and colleagues recently demonstrated that librarian-led instruction can positively impact resource selection.[16] Thus a key task for medical librarians is increasing learner awareness of the available resources and helping them develop and hone resource selection skills. A variety of common information needs are described below, and resources that are useful in each situation are highlighted.

EMBARRASSED-TO-ASK QUESTIONS

Medical trainees are not the only ones reluctant to ask questions; it is common among all levels of learners.[17] However, reluctance to ask questions out of fear or embarrassment may be more common in the often fiercely competitive realm of medical education.[18] The perception among students and residents that they "should" know something or that they are the only one among their peers who does not know—regardless of the accuracy of that perception—creates a major barrier to asking questions. Quick reference titles, such as Ferri's *Clinical Advisor* and *Quick Medical Diagnosis and Treatment*, are ideally suited as a first reference for those too embarrassed to ask. These texts are designed to provide high-level overviews, including core information on clinical features, diagnosis, treatment, and prognosis for thousands of diseases and conditions. Their content is formatted in bullet points, rather than long-form paragraphs, making it easier to read and digest the material quickly and ideal for quick look-ups on the wards.

IN-DEPTH BACKGROUND KNOWLEDGE

For medical students tasked with putting together a short presentation on a disease or condition or interns treating a patient with a comorbid condition they have never encountered, textbook aggregator sites—including Access-Medicine, ClinicalKey, and LWW Health Library—are excellent resources. These sites each feature hundreds of different texts, eliminating the need for lengthy consideration of which book might contain the needed information. Textbooks provide in-depth information suitable for a thorough introduction or refresher on a topic without providing excessive details about nuanced treatment and management decisions.

AT THE POINT OF CARE

Questions that arise at the point of care (PoC) vary widely and pertain to myriad topics including symptoms, diagnostic tests, drug choice, drug dosing and administration, management, and prognosis.[19] Drug monographs and databases such as Micromedex and Lexicomp are the most effective resources for answering questions about drug dosing, administration, side effects, adverse effects, and other questions related to prescription medications.

For other types of point-of-care questions, clinical information summary tools, primarily UpToDate and DynaMed, are typically the best resources. Clinical information summary tools, sometimes called clinical evidence summary resources or PoC resources, are best thought of as encyclopedias for health-care professionals. These resources aim to provide current, comprehensive coverage of the clinical presentation, diagnosis, treatment, and prognosis for thousands of conditions. Clinical information summary tools feature nuanced information on treatment and management decisions and excel at answering this kind of information need. Consistent anecdotal feedback from learners and practicing clinicians indicates that UpToDate is the preferred resource at the PoC because of the way its entries are organized and formatted. Though not appropriate for occasions that call for detailed knowledge of the strength of the evidence, UpToDate is the best choice for quick look-ups at the PoC.

A DEEP DIVE

While a quick look-up on the floor may be sufficient to proceed with a decision related to patient care, learning the why behind common practices is an important aspect of medical education. Why is this diagnostic test used? Why is that drug prescribed? Why is this therapy superior to that therapy in this patient population? Often the questioner will explicitly ask, "What is the evidence for . . . ?" or "What is the strength of the evidence for . . . ?" Morning report is one of the most common forums for these types of questions.

For these occasions, DynaMed+ and pre-appraised resources such as ACP Journal Club and AAP Grand Rounds are essential. DynaMed+ features the main conclusion of a study in a headline-like format, followed by robust detailed information about the study, including study design, setting, methodological limitations, and whether results were significant. It includes key information from study results such as likelihood ratios and number needed to treat (NNT). Another feature that makes DynaMed+ useful for deep-dive information needs is that it provides evidence grading both at the recommendation level and the individual study level. This helps users evaluate the strength of the overall body of literature on a topic as well as the quality of the individual studies.

While DynaMed is excellent for gaining an understanding of the scope and strength of the evidence on a given topic, pre-appraised resources provide users with detailed information on a single study. Pre-appraised resources "include only studies and reviews that are more likely to be methodologically sound and clinically relevant."[20] Drawing from this pool of studies, experts offer a robust critical appraisal, including the highlights and lowlights of the study's methodology and limitations to generalizability. Because only studies of higher quality that have potentially practice-changing implications are included, these sites have only a few thousand entries. This makes them easier and more manageable to search and review results compared to large bibliographic databases. Pre-appraised resources can be used alone or in combination with Dynamed for users seeking in-depth knowledge of the available evidence.

WHEN TO USE AND WHEN NOT TO USE

Table 9.1 summarizes information from this section about which resources are most useful for different situations and information needs. The table also includes suggestions about when these resources would not be useful or appropriate.

BEYOND ASK AND ACQUIRE—LEVERAGING OUR ROLES

The focus of the chapter so far has been on the *ask* and *acquire* steps in the EBM cycle and the librarian's role in instruction on these topics. As has been reported, librarians typically play a less active role in educating clinical learners on the *appraise* and *apply* steps,[21] though this is not universally true[22] and there have been calls for librarians to develop their skills in this regard to allow them to become more involved in the full cycle of EBM teaching.[23] New professional development opportunities to address this need, particularly on the topic of critical appraisal, have recently been developed. These include a continuing education course, CE302 Teaching Critical Appraisal Skills, that was offered for the first time at the Medical Library Association 2019 Annual Meeting, and the Critical Appraisal Institute for Librarians online course that was offered for the first time in the spring of 2019.[24]

These efforts are laudable, but it will take time for these educational efforts to permeate among health science librarians. In the meanwhile, librarians can leverage existing roles outside the instruction arena to support the development of critical appraisal and application of evidence to patient care in clinical learners.

Table 9.1. When to Use Tipsheet

Resource	When to Use	Not Useful	Mobile App Available
Quick reference texts (e.g., Quick Medical Dx and Tx)	• You need a super quick intro or refresher on a condition • Things you feel like you "should" know	• When you need detailed information • When you're asked to cite primary literature	Quick Medical Dx and Tx available on Access Medicine app
Access Medicine	• Your attending asks you to put together a five-minute presentation on a medical condition • You need a deep dive/refresher on a condition your patient has	• On the wards • When you're asked to cite primary literature	Yes
UpToDate	• Quick look-ups for your patients • Specific information to make plans for patients	• As sole source of information • When you're asked to cite primary literature	Yes
DynaMed+	• You need a deep dive into the evidence • First step when attending asks you, "What's the evidence/strength of evidence for X?"	• Quick look-up on the wards • Dosing specifics • Background reading	Yes
Pre-appraised resources (e.g., ACP Journal Club)	• Want to get an in-depth look at one study plus a general sense of where it fits in with existing literature • Want to discuss a specific paper on rounds but do not have time to fully appraise yourself	• Quick look-up on the wards • Background reading	No

CURRICULUM DEVELOPMENT

Multiple publications have documented the involvement of librarians in curriculum development.[25] A 2015 study by Maggio and colleagues describes the varied roles that health science librarians play in curriculum development:

> As curricular designers, participants developed content, determined content delivery methods, created supporting materials, identified subject matter experts, such as epidemiologists and clinical faculty, and sequenced EBM sessions within the larger curriculum. In this role, participants discussed their familiarity with the overall medical school curriculum. Participants described the importance of designing EBM curriculum to be situated appropriately to ensure that learners had context for understanding the relevance of EBM to clinical practice.[26]

Of particular interest is librarian involvement in content development and sequencing. Librarians can use these roles to advocate for the inclusion of important topics in the curriculum and participate in content and instructional design for sessions that cover these topics.

RESOURCE CURATION

While many novel roles for medical librarians—some of which are detailed elsewhere in this volume—have emerged in recent years, curating and suggesting resources in the form of subject guides has long been a core role and skill set for librarians.[27] The advent of the widely adopted LibGuides online content creation and management system has made it easier than ever for librarians to curate a selection of targeted, high-quality resources on a given topic.[28]

Librarians can put their curriculum development and resource curation expertise to good use for many purposes. Here we suggest two EBM-adjacent topics of particular importance: clinical communication skills and the shortcomings of the medical literature. We recommend that health science librarians use their skills to increase knowledge and awareness of these topics.

CLINICAL COMMUNICATION SKILLS

Beyond finding and utilizing information themselves, the importance of clinicians sharing information with patients and engaging them in the decision-making process is increasingly being recognized.[29] The ability to communicate effectively is an essential, prerequisite skill required for clinicians to be able to learn about a patient's values and preferences in order to apply these to their care. Shared decision-making has been shown to improve patient outcomes[30] and may have a role to play in minimizing overprescribing.[31] However, communicating about the availability and quality of evidence, benefits and harms, and clinical uncertainty is challenging. Learning to elicit patient preferences and values is another difficult skill to master.

Clinical decision aids are designed to help patients engage in the medical decision-making process in concert with their health-care provider. Per the Commonwealth Fund's definition, "Decision aids such as educational literature, videos, or Web-based tools are designed to help patients prepare for these conversations by weighing the potential benefits, risks, and uncertainties of a medical procedure."[32] A number of high-quality decision aids exist, but they are not currently widely used in clinical practice.[33] Two particularly highly regarded creators of decision aids are the Mayo Clinic and the Ottawa Hospital. The excellent tools provided by these organizations have the added benefit of being freely available. There are a number of additional resources currently available, both free and licensed, that libraries can evaluate, license (if required), and recommend.

Clinical medical librarians can help increase awareness of and access to these tools and, in so doing, help increase uptake of this practice by the next generation of physicians. Creating a finding guide on the library's website with basic information about and links to high-quality decision aids is a potentially impactful way that medical librarians can help clinical learners become strong communicators. Additionally, librarians can leverage their role in curriculum development to suggest that education and training on this topic be woven in to the EBM curriculum.

LIMITATIONS OF EBM

While equipping students with EBM skills is crucial, it is also important that we educate learners about the shortcomings of the medical literature—and by extension of EBM—so that learners have a realistic understanding of both its advantages and potential pitfalls. Problems with the medical literature are well documented.[34] Prevalent issues include the influence of pharmaceutical funding on research outcomes[35] and the influence of the pharmaceutical industry more broadly.[36] Career-related concerns and the publish-or-perish culture have also been identified as culprits.[37] These issues extend beyond individual studies into clinical practice guidelines.[38] Educating clinical learners on how to acquire and utilize evidence without alerting them to the shortcomings of the medical literature does them a disservice. Librarians can and must exercise their roles in curriculum development and resource curation to help educate clinical learners on these topics.

CONCLUSION

Health science librarians have long played a role in educating clinical learners. In this chapter we have reviewed the librarian's well-established role in instruction, particularly with regard to asking clinical questions and acquiring best evidence, and we have highlighted important considerations for librarians as they go about this work. Heightened awareness of common challenges in clinical question formulation and resource selection will allow librarians to better address these issues during instruction sessions. By suggesting situationally appropriate resources, librarians can help clinical learners become more effective information seekers. Beyond the realm of instruction, librarians can utilize their involvement in curriculum development to advocate for the inclusion of important and sometimes overlooked topics and use their skills at resource curation to create engaging, relevant subject guides to further aid in the education of clinical learners on these topics.

ACKNOWLEDGMENTS

I gratefully acknowledge and thank Dr. Andrew Coyle, assistant professor of medicine and associate program director of the Internal Medicine Residency at the Icahn School of Medicine at Mount Sinai, with whom I collaborated to create the When to Use Tipsheet.

NOTES

1. P. Glasziou, A. Burls, and R. Gilbert, "Evidence-Based Medicine and the Medical Curriculum," *BMJ* 337 (2008).

2. D. Grahame-Smith, "Evidence-Based Medicine: Socratic Dissent," *BMJ: British Medical Journal* 310, no. 6987 (1995); R. I. Horwitz, "The Dark Side of Evidence-Based Medicine," *Cleve Clin J Med* 63, no. 6 (1996); M. Tonelli, "The Philosophical Limits of Evidence-Based Medicine" (1998); S. E. Straus and F. A. McAlister, "Evidence-Based Medicine: A Commentary on Common Criticisms," *Cmaj* 163, no. 7 (2000).

3. Liaison Committee on Medical Education, "Functions and Structure of a Medical School—Standards for Accreditation of Medical Education Programs Leading to the Md Degree" (Washington, D.C., 2018); Accreditation Council for Graduate Medical Education, "Acgme Common Program Requirements" (2017).

4. C. S. Scherrer and J. L. Dorsch, "The Evolving Role of the Librarian in Evidence-Based Medicine," *Bull Med Libr Assoc* 87, no. 3 (1999); P. Li and L. Wu, "Supporting Evidence-Based Medicine: A Survey of U.S. Medical Librarians," *Med Ref Serv Q* 30, no. 4 (2011); L. A. Maggio, N. Durieux, and N. H. Tannery, "Librarians in Evidence-Based Medicine Curricula: A Qualitative Study of Librarian Roles, Training, and Desires for Future Development," *Med Ref Serv Q* 34, no. 4 (2015).

5. A. Schwartz and G. Millam, "A Web-Based Library Consult Service for Evidence-Based Medicine: Technical Development," *BMC Med Inform Decis Mak* 6 (2006); M. Moore, "Teaching Physicians to Make Informed Decisions in the Face of Uncertainty: Librarians and Informaticians on the Health Care Team," *Acad Med* 86, no. 11 (2011); M. J. Kash, "Teaching Evidence-Based Medicine in the Era of Point-of-Care Databases: The Case of the Giant Blad-

der Stone," *Med Ref Serv Q* 35, no. 2 (2016); A. Minuti et al., "Librarians Flip for Students: Teaching Searching Skills to Medical Students Using a Flipped Classroom Approach," *Med Ref Serv Q* 37, no. 2 (2018); L. E. Herrmann et al., "Integrating a Clinical Librarian to Increase Trainee Application of Evidence-Based Medicine on Patient Family-Centered Rounds," *Acad Pediatr* 17, no. 3 (2017); L. D. Gruppen, G. K. Rana, and T. S. Arndt, "A Controlled Comparison Study of the Efficacy of Training Medical Students in Evidence-Based Medicine Literature Searching Skills," *Acad Med* 80, no. 10 (2005).

6. V. Moyer, "Weighing the Evidence: Pico Questions: What Are They, and Why Bother?" *AAP Grand Rounds* 19, no. 1 (2008); D. O'Sullivan et al., "Using Pico to Align Medical Evidence with MDs Decision Making Models," *Stud Health Technol Inform* 192 (2013).

7. K. Lloyd et al., "Analysis of Clinical Uncertainties by Health Professionals and Patients: An Example from Mental Health," *BMC Med Inform Decis Mak* 9, no. 34 (2009).

8. Moyer, "Weighing the Evidence"; S. E. Straus et al., *Evidence-Based Medicine: How to Practice and Teach EBM* (Edinburgh: Elsevier, 2019); Centre for Evidence Based Medicine, "Asking Focused Questions," www.cebm.net/2014/06/asking-focused-questions; McMaster Univeristy Health Science Library, "Nursing: Forming Questions," https://hslmcmaster.libguides.com/nursing/questions; G. Del Fiol, T. E. Workman, and P. N. Gorman, "Clinical Questions Raised by Clinicians at the Point of Care: A Systematic Review," *JAMA internal medicine* 174, no. 5 (2014).

9. Biomarkers Definitions Working Group, "Biomarkers and Surrogate Endpoints: Preferred Definitions and Conceptual Framework," *Clinical Pharmacology & Therapeutics* 69, no. 3 (2001).

10. H. C. Bucher et al., "Surrogate Outcomes," in *Users' Guides to the Medical Literature: A Manual for Evidence-Based Clinical Practice,* 3rd ed., ed. Gordon Guyatt et al. (New York: McGraw-Hill Education, 2015).

11. Maggio, Durieux, and Tannery, "Librarians in Evidence-Based Medicine Curricula."

12. A. V. Epps and M. S. Nelson, "One-Shot or Embedded? Assessing Different Delivery Timing for Information Resources Relevant to Assignments," *Evidence Based Library and Information Practice* 8, no. 1 (2013); A. Conway, "One-Shot Library Instruction Sessions May Not Increase Student Use of Academic Journals or Diversity of Sources," *J Evidence Based Library and Information Practice* 10, no. 4 (2015).

13. M. MacEachern et al., "Librarian Integration in a Four-Year Medical School Curriculum: A Timeline," *Medical Reference Services Quarterly* 31, no. 1 (2012); S. Clifton and P. Jo, "A Journey Worth Taking: Exploring a Hybrid Embedded Library Instruction Model through Three Distinct Cases," *Med Ref Serv Q* 35, no. 3 (2016); E. M. Geyer and D. E. Irish, "Isolated to Integrated: An Evolving Medical Informatics Curriculum," *Med Ref Serv Q* 27, no. 4 (2008).

14. P. Wyer et al., "Teachers' Guides to the Users' Guides," in *Users' Guides to the Medical Literature: A Manual for Evidence-Based Clinical Practice,* 3rd ed., ed. Gordon Guyatt et al. (New York: McGraw-Hill Education, 2015).

15. E. A. Sastre et al., "Teaching Evidence-Based Medicine: Impact on Students' Literature Use and Inpatient Clinical Documentation," *Medical Teacher* 33, no. 6 (2011).

16. J. K. Gaines et al., "Partnering to Analyze Selection of Resources by Medical Students for Case-Based Small Group Learning: A Collaboration between Librarians and Medical Educators," *Med Ref Serv Q* 37, no. 3 (2018).

17. J. T. Dillon, "A Norm against Student Questions," *The Clearing House: A Journal of Educational Strategies, Issues and Ideas* 55, no. 3 (1981); W. J. Lammers to Faculty Focus, 2017, www.facultyfocus.com/articles/effective-classroom-management/wont-ask-us-help.

18. Anonymous to KevinMD, October 21, 2016, www.kevinmd.com/blog/2016/10/stop-competition-medical-school.html; J. M. Sutton-Klein, "I'm Less Competitive Than You: Competition on the Wards Takes Our Focus Away from Patients," *Student BMJ* (2015).

19. Del Fiol, Workman, and Gorman, "Clinical Questions Raised"; J. W. Ely et al., "Analysis of Questions Asked by Family Doctors Regarding Patient Care," *Bmj* 319, no. 7206 (1999); J. W. Ely et al., "A Taxonomy of Generic Clinical Questions: Classification Study," *Bmj* 321, no. 7258 (2000).

20. T. Agoritsas et al., "Finding Current Best Evidence," in *Users' Guides to the Medical Literature: A Manual for Evidence-Based Clinical Practice,* 3rd ed., ed. Gordon Guyatt et al. (New York: McGraw-Hill Education, 2015).

21. Maggio, Durieux, and Tannery, "Librarians in Evidence-Based Medicine Curricula."

22. Scherrer and Dorsch, "The Evolving Role of the Librarian"; M. Maden-Jenkins, "Healthcare Librarians and the Delivery of Critical Appraisal Training: Attitudes, Level of Involvement and Support," *Health Info Libr J* 27, no. 4 (2010).

23. J. Costello, "Updating Professional Development for Medical Librarians to Improve Our Evidence-Based Medicine and Information Literacy Instruction," *J Med Libr Assoc* 106, no. 3 (2018).

24. The author was on the Critical Appraisal Institute for Librarians planning committee.

25. I. Kovar-Gough, "Taking Chances: A New Librarian and Curriculum Redesign," *Med Ref Serv Q* 36, no. 2 (2017); J. M. Muellenbach et al., "Integrating Information Literacy and Evidence-Based Medicine Content within a New School of Medicine Curriculum: Process and Outcome," *Med Ref Serv Q* 37 (2018); M. L. Klem and P. M. Weiss, "Evidence-Based Resources and the Role of Librarians in Developing Evidence-Based Practice Curricula," *J Prof Nurs* 21, no. 6 (2005); K. Zeblisky, R. A. Birr, and A. M. Sjursen Guerrero, "Effecting Change in an Evidence-Based Medicine Curriculum: Librarians' Role in a Pediatric Residency Program," *Med Ref Serv Q* 34, no. 3 (2015).

26. Maggio, Durieux, and Tannery, "Librarians in Evidence-Based Medicine Curricula."

27. C. Dahl, "Electronic Pathfinders in Academic Libraries: An Analysis of Their Content and Form," *College and Research Libraries* 62, no. 3 (2001); R. Jackson and L. Pellack, "Internet Subject Guides in Academic Libraries: An Analysis of Contents, Practices, and Opinions," *Ref Use Serv Q* (2004); L. G. Adebonojo, "Libguides: Customizing Subject Guides for Individual Courses," *College and Undergraduate Libraries* 17, no. 4 (2010); J. Jansen et al., "Too Much Medicine in Older People? Deprescribing through Shared Decision Making," *BMJ (Online)* 353 (2016).

28. L. Vileno, "From Paper to Electronic, the Evolution of Pathfinders: A Review of the Literature," *Reference Services Review* 35, no. 3 (2007); N. R. Glassman and K. Sorensen, "From Pathfinders to Subject Guides: One Library's Experience with Libguides," *Journal of Electronic Resources in Medical Libraries* 7, no. 4 (2010).

29. T. R. Fried, "Shared Decision Making—Finding the Sweet Spot," *New England Journal of Medicine* 374, no. 2 (2016); M. J. Barry and S. Edgman-Levitan, "Shared Decision Making—the Pinnacle of Patient-Centered Care," *New England Journal of Medicine* 366, no. 9 (2012).

30. E. A. G. Joosten et al., "Systematic Review of the Effects of Shared Decision-Making on Patient Satisfaction, Treatment Adherence and Health Status," *Psychotherapy and Psychosomatics* 77, no. 4 (2008); L. Aubree Shay and J. E. Lafata, "Where Is the Evidence? A Systematic Review of Shared Decision Making and Patient Outcomes," *Medical Decision Making* 35, no. 1 (2015).

31. Jansen et al., "Too Much Medicine in Older People?"

32. M. Hostetter and S. Klein, "Helping Patients Make Better Treatment Choices with Decision Aids," The Commonwealth Fund, www.commonwealthfund.org/publications/newsletter-article/helping-patients-make-better-treatment-choices-decision-aids.

33. D. Stacey et al., "Decision Aids for People Facing Health Treatment or Screening Decisions," *Cochrane Database of Systematic Reviews,* no. 4 (2017).

34. D. G. Altman, "The Scandal of Poor Medical Research" (British Medical Journal Publishing Group, 1994); J. P. A. Ioannidis, "Why Most Published Research Findings Are False," *PLoS Medicine* 2, no. 8 (2005); J. P. A. Ioannidis, "Contradicted and Initially Stronger Effects in Highly Cited Clinical Research," *Journal of the American Medical Association* 294, no. 2 (2005); B. Goldacre, *Bad Science: Quacks, Hacks, and Big Pharma Flacks* (Toronto: Emblem, 2011).

35. J. Lexchin et al., "Pharmaceutical Industry Sponsorship and Research Outcome and Quality: Systematic Review," *BMJ (Clinical research ed.)* 326, no. 7400 (2003); S. S. Chopra, "Industry Funding of Clinical Trials: Benefit or Bias?," *JAMA* 290, no. 1 (2003).

36. B. Goldacre, *Bad Pharma: How Drug Companies Mislead Doctors and Harm Patients*, 1st American ed. (New York: Faber and Faber, 2013).

37. M. S. Anderson et al., "The Perverse Effects of Competition on Scientists' Work and Relationships," *Sci Eng Ethics* 13, no. 4 (2007); D. Fanelli, R. Costas, and V. Larivière, "Misconduct Policies, Academic Culture and Career Stage, Not Gender or Pressures to Publish, Affect Scientific Integrity," *PloS one* 10, no. 6 (2015); S. L. Norris et al., "Conflict of Interest Disclosures for Clinical Practice Guidelines in the National Guideline Clearinghouse," *PLoS One* 7, no. 11 (2012).

38. A. R. Amiri et al., "Does Source of Funding and Conflict of Interest Influence the Outcome and Quality of Spinal Research?" *Spine J* 14, no. 2 (2014); L. Cosgrove et al., "Conflict of Interest Policies and Industry Relationships of Guideline Development Group Members: A Cross-Sectional Study of Clinical Practice Guidelines for Depression," *Account Res* 24, no. 2 (2017); H. C. Sox, "Conflict of Interest in Practice Guidelines Panels," *JAMA* 317, no. 17 (2017).

Chapter Ten

A Clinical Medical Library Internship

Keith C. Mages and Becky Baltich Nelson

Lack of available specialized training for aspirant clinical medical librarians (CML) and institutions looking to hire them is a major challenge. Masters of Library Science (MLS) programs offering tracks or specializations focused on health librarianship are scarce, and those focused on clinical medical librarianship even more so. Some MLS programs describe health librarianship courses in their catalogs, but those courses are not guaranteed to be offered with regularity.[1] Despite being engaged in point-of-care clinical roles since the 1970s,[2] librarians often utilize on-the-job training rather than formal educational opportunities to learn specialized skills required for these positions. Because many librarians' first degree is in arts and humanities, they often lack knowledge of medical terminology and jargon used in healthcare settings.[3] Recent survey responses revealed that librarians with a first degree in a scientific area saw the immediate benefit and applicability of their subject knowledge area and that it instilled confidence in their abilities in the CML role.[4]

A few CML internships or residencies have been developed to ameliorate the paucity of CML educational opportunities. Notable among these is the Vanderbilt Eskind Biomedical Library program, which trains librarians in the clinical setting and focuses on evidence-based medicine, search and filter skills, formal university coursework and building subject-area expertise.[5] For the most part, training remains limited, and in 2015 almost 70 percent of surveyed CMLs reported they were self-taught. Respondents described engaging in self-directed activities such as reading medical journals, learning medical terminology and laboratory tests and values, studying evidence-based medicine practices, and taking professional development courses when possible. They expressed a desire for mentorship and topical training to provide maximum value to their patient-care teams.[6]

Administrators at the Samuel J. Wood Library of Weill Cornell Medicine (WCM) in New York recognized the extent of this issue during a faculty search for a new clinical medical librarian. The applicant pool contained excellent librarians, but few had explicit experience or training in clinical medical librarianship. After hiring a candidate, the library director and CML team helped bridge the gap between library programs and entry-level jobs by developing an internship program to prepare new and soon-to-be librarians to assume CML roles and responsibilities.

In 2016, WCM initiated a one-year paid internship for an advanced student enrolled in an American Library Association accredited library and information science graduate program to work as a clinical medical librarian intern (CMLI or intern). The intern assists the CML team in providing biomedical research, information management, and instructional services to clinical and academic communities of Weill Cornell Medicine (WCM), New York–Presbyterian Hospital (NYP), and affiliates. The CMLI supports and enhances clinical practices, outreach activities, and training initiatives of WCM and its constituents. As of 2019, three interns completed the program and are now employed in hospital or academic health sciences libraries. This chapter describes the components and structure of the WCM program and discusses plans to develop a robust program evaluation.

COMPONENTS AND STRUCTURE

The WCM internship provides CMLIs a variety of learning experiences and activities that are curricular and professional in nature. Curricular activities provide instruction on the fundamentals of CML roles and responsibilities, while professional activities focus on acquiring practical knowledge and gaining experience in a variety of clinical health-care environments. The professional component of the program consumes more CMLI time, but the curricular component is equally weighted. Successfully managing a calendar and juggling projects, deadlines, and meetings is critical in bustling academic medical centers. The supervising CML creates a team calendar to help the CMLI organize his or her time. The CMLI learns to visualize and prioritize commitments, as their calendar quickly fills with online coursework, seminar-style discussion groups, and a variety of clinical duties, including attending morning report and joining residents and students on clinical rounds. During weekly meetings with their CML supervisor, interns check in to report routine matters, ask questions, and seek advice or just talk.

The CMLI curriculum component, anchored by an asynchronous learning experience centered on monthly modules and housed in WCM's online learning management software, is a familiar tableau for new library school graduates.[7] CMLIs participate in a monthly seminar-style discussion group at the conclusion of each module and are expected to identify and utilize important health science resources and discuss issues raised by content materials.

Course objectives for the CMLI curriculum include:

- identifying and utilizing electronic library resources available at Samuel J. Wood library;
- discussing components of evidence-based medicine, including:

  - differentiating between background and foreground questions;

- discussing the librarian's role in consumer health and patient education, including:

  - identifying and evaluating patient education resources;

- engaging in health literacy discussions;
- identifying funding opportunities in health science librarianship;
- understanding the systematic review process including the librarian's role;
- recognizing the librarian's role in the publishing process, including:

  - librarian scholarship and
  - knowledge of predatory publishers;

- appreciating the librarian's role in the electronic health record; and
- identifying major career resources available to health sciences librarians, including:

  - developing a professional CV.

Monthly Modules

Twelve monthly modules consisting of videos, journal articles, and activities on a variety of topics relevant to contemporary issues in medical librarianship comprise the curriculum. A module is made available at 12:00 a.m. on the first of every month. CMLIs have protected time to work through the online curriculum; we chose to stagger access to each module to ensure interns do not feel pressured to work ahead of schedule but to utilize their protected time for thoughtful analysis of assigned content instead. The modules are:

1. Clinical Medical Librarian Skill-Building Coursework and Reference Materials
2. Key Biomedical Databases

3. Evidence Based Medicine
4. Consumer Health and Patient Education
5. Health Literacy
6. Scholarly Communication & Predatory Publishing
7. Systematic Reviews, Meta Analyses and Other Reviews
8. Selection, Management, and Delivery of Health Information Resources
9. Research and Funding Opportunities in Health Sciences Libraries
10. Electronic and Personal Health Records
11. Career Development
12. Future of Health Care & Health Sciences Librarianship

CMLIs are encouraged to keep track of questions and comments while working in the modules and bring those to the seminar discussion, a monthly meeting hosted by the CML supervisor and attended by the entire CML team. CMLIs are encouraged to provide feedback on each module's assigned learning materials during the discussion. The CML supervisor promotes thoughtful dialogue and actively seeks feedback on how the intern experienced each component of the module. To encourage active participation, we ask interns to identify a topical, relevant resource that corresponds to the particular subject of each module. The resource can be any format.

Core Information Resources

"Core Information Resource" quizzes are included in most modules. A Qualtrics-generated quiz consisting of five to ten fill-in-the-blank or multiple-choice questions test CMLI knowledge of where to locate information from a variety of library sources, including print. Most of our quizzes highlight texts of particular relevance to specific medical fields. In recognition of the importance of seminal textbooks and the suggestion of our library director, the CML team consulted the most recent Brandon/Hill Selected List of Print Books and Journals to identify classic core medical texts.[8] The following medical specialty areas are highlighted in select modules: pediatrics, internal medicine, evidence-based medicine, surgery/anesthesiology, cardiology, neurology, and oncology. The intern must answer subject-knowledge questions generated by members of the CML team using the most recent version of identified textbooks.

Special Projects

CMLIs complete three special projects during the year: (1) present a consumer health/patient information session to a local seniors group, (2) identify a potential funding opportunity for CML services and write a one-page prospectus for the project, and (3) identify a potential job opportunity and create a cover letter that articulates how their experiences meet the advertised needs.

Module 2: Key Biomedical Databases

A detailed examination of the Key Biomedical Databases module, an overview of teaching resources, core information resources quiz questions, specific activities assigned, and seminar discussion points follows. It is our hope this information may helpful to other medical libraries considering launching their own CMLI programs. As the module was developed specifically for WCM and NYP, not all of the content may be of relevance to other institutions. We encourage readers to modify the following content however they see fit.

The Key Databases module introduces CMLIs to some of the most commonly used databases at WCM and features vendor-produced YouTube videos and instructions for PubMed, Ovid MEDLINE, Ovid EMBASE, and CINAHL. CMLIs read two articles on database searching that approach the topic from the clinician's viewpoint. Kelly et al.'s *So Many Databases, Such Little Clarity* offers a unique glimpse into how clinicians conceptualize the utility of biomedical databases.[9] It is especially fascinating for its perspective into clinicians' understanding of journal indexing and searching practices. DeGroote et al's *Information-Seeking Behavior and the Use of Online Resources* evaluates online databases most commonly used by clinicians.[10] DeGroote's article not only reveals clinician's database preference but also includes a provocative interpretation of ways librarians can apply this knowledge.

Core Information Resources in Internal Medicine

Sample Quiz Questions (Please reference page numbers with your answers.)

1. Using *Andreoli and Carpenter's Cecil Essentials of Medicine*, 9th edition, define *acute liver failure* (ALF).[11] What older term does ALF replace?
2. Using this same resource, identify the organ systems that may be impacted by systemic lupus erythematosus (SLE).
3. Locate *Harrison's Principles of Internal Medicine*, 20th edition.[12] Using this resource, identify the four broad domains fundamental to the provision of quality palliative care and end-of-life care.
4. Using this same resource, define Hashimoto's thyroiditis. What other diseases must be ruled out when considering differential diagnosis?
5. How does the most recent edition of the *Washington Manual of Medical Therapeutics* advise clinicians to treat clostridium difficile-associated diarrhea?[13]

Seminar discussions for this module focus on the intern's general understanding and thoughts on the utility and functionality of each biomedical database, offer discourse on assigned readings, and provide an article investigating some aspect of clinician searching. We end this session with a review of their monthly quiz results.

PROFESSIONAL ROLE DEVELOPMENT

The CMLI's curricular course content is extensive, but the majority of intern time is consumed by professional tasks and responsibilities. By the third month of the internship, CMLIs are usually functioning like any other CML and balancing clinical and reference responsibilities, teaching expectations, research pursuits, and continuing educational experiences within a busy schedule. Before taking on these responsibilities, interns are on-boarded in a systematic fashion.

Upon arrival, each new CMLI is introduced to the various divisions and services of the Samuel J. Wood Library. Over the course of the first few weeks, CMLIs meet with representatives from all library departments during thirty-minute orientation sessions where the intern meets other library staff members and learns about the library layout and procedures. The intern meets hospital and outpatient clinical clients during a month long "shadow" period while accompanying a senior CML team member on rounds. The transition from shadowing to attending clinical rounds on their own is gradual.

Initially, interns observe and take notes. After clinical sessions, the accompanying CML team member meets with the CMLI to discuss clinical questions, possible databases to search, and best search strategies to answer questions. The CML performs a search, selects articles, and sends the results to the clinician. The CMLI observes the search method and communication style of the CML. The CMLI is encouraged to offer his or her thoughts and perspectives on database selection and search strategy as time passes. Although still accompanied by the CML, the CMLI usually takes the lead with clinical teams during the second month. The CML checks intern search strategies and drafts of communication prior to dissemination of results to the clinical teams. When the CML determines the CMLI's search and interpersonal communication skills are consistent and of high quality, the intern can "fly solo."

Clinical and Reference

The CML team supports education and clinical practice of residents in the Department of Medicine (DOM) at WCM/NYP. Attending the DOM's morning report is one of the first clinical experiences for a CMLI. Thrice weekly DOM residents at morning report discuss interesting or educational clinical cases. CMLs take notes throughout these presentations, record any unanswered explicit or implicit questions, and follow up with the chief residents at the conclusion of morning report. CMLs search for clinical information and email results to the chief resident or upload annotated PDFs to a joint F1000 Workspace folder. The method of delivery depends on preferences of the specific chief resident.

CMLs at WCM also liaise with the Department of Pediatrics (Pediatrics) at NYP/WCM. Once a week, CMLs join two provider teams during family-centered rounds. Teams are comprised of an attending physician, pediatric residents, medical students, a clinical pharmacist, and pharmacy students. The CML supports evidence-based practice by answering clinical questions at the point of care and providing follow-up literature searches to enhance resident comprehension of identified topics. CMLs also provide consumer health information to any patient and/or family member in need of assistance. Consumer information requests may be prompted by the attending physician or senior resident or initiated by the CML themselves. In these situations, the CML stays with the patient after the clinical team leaves to assess patient and family needs.

Teaching

CMLIs participate in the full range of teaching opportunities available to WCM librarians. Opportunities include teaching clinical question formulation and PICO search building to medical students, EBP methods and resources during neurology clerkships, overviews of systematic reviews to medical residents, and faculty/staff library orientations. CMLIs may teach these classes in tandem with another librarian or lead them independently. CMLIs are also encouraged to identify a topic and lead a "Tech Tuesdays" session. Each Tuesday of the month, WCM library hosts Tech Tuesdays, a thirty-minute showcase at 12:00 p.m., to highlight various tools and software available to members of the WCM/NYP community.

In addition to teaching students, faculty, and staff, CMLIs are also tasked with teaching a selected consumer health or patient education topic at our consumer health library, the Myra Mahon Patient Resource Center (PRC). This experience provides a valuable opportunity to work with community seniors and challenges CMLIs to adjust their teaching style to fit the needs of a unique participant group. To further understand and appreciate the needs of local community members, CMLIs are also encouraged to assist during the other occurrences of the PRC seminar series, supporting registration, audio-visual, and promotional needs.

Research Participation

Research is one of the core components of WCM's mission. Accordingly, CMLIs are provided with opportunities to contribute to institutional scholarship. Each CMLI participates in the library's systematic review service. When requested by research teams, the service partners a WCM librarian with the requesting systematic review team. Over the course of this collaboration, librarians and CMLIs may:

- help define a research question;
- assist in development and registration of an SR protocol;
- recommend specific databases and other resources to be searched;
- identify database-specific search strategies, using a combination of appropriate keywords and controlled vocabulary;
- conduct literature searches;
- pull references from bibliographies and hand searching procedures;
- deliver results into a bibliographic management tool such as EndNote or Mendeley, or into SR management software such as Covidence;
- perform search updates, as needed; and
- suggest relevant journals to explore publication options.[14]

This service is free of charge to all NYP/WCM faculty, staff, and students, and librarians (including CMLIs) are given author credit on all resulting presentations and publications. As with all other programs in which they participate, CMLIs collaborate with another librarian before moving to a more independent role.

CMLIs are also encouraged to participate in other research or special projects. In the past, CMLIs have engaged in personal archival and special collections research projects, collaborated on librarian-led systematic reviews, and participated in the development of materials in support of funded library grants.

Conference Support

CMLIs are provided with financial support to attend training sessions and professional conferences. To supplement their understanding and comfort with the systematic review process, all CMLIs participate in the University of Pittsburgh Health Sciences Library System's Systematic Review Workshop: The Nuts and Bolts for Librarians. Additionally, CMLIs receive financial support to attend the annual conference of the Medical Library Association. Each of these experiences is intended to enhance CMLI skillset development, as well as to provide valuable professional networking opportunities.

PROGRAM EVALUATION

Effective evaluation of any library program provides administrators with information needed to justify continued support of the program. This is certainly applicable for internship programs that require significant staff time and financial resources for professional development activities and salaried internship positions. Program evaluation is another administrative cost of an internship that is necessary to ensure the experience is valuable to the intern's career growth and trajectory and that learned skills provide value to the profession and supporting institution.[15]

Currently, evaluation for our program happens informally throughout the duration of the internship. Supervisors and the intern meet regularly to discuss expectations, experiences, and progress. These meetings allow both parties to determine what is working and what modifications may be required to meet needs on each side. At the end of the internship, a final debriefing between intern and supervisor and an exit interview with the institution's human resources department occurs. Thus far, feedback from the interns and tracking post-internship job placement are our best indicators of success.

We plan to implement a more robust evaluation system for the CMLI program. Currently we are researching existing evaluation methodologies such as the National Network of Libraries of Medicine's Collecting and Analyzing Evaluation Data.[16] We are considering a three-pronged approach to evaluate the intern and program.

- Step 1: a survey of the intern at the end of the internship. Survey questions may ask the intern to rate different facets of the experience, indicate if they would recommend the internship to others, and offer suggestions for future interns and suggestions to improve the program. Data will be tracked over time and used by the CML team to continually refine the program.
- Step 2: intern completes a supervisor evaluation form at the middle and end of the internship. The form seeks feedback for the supervisor to aid in designing training and developing a relationship tailored to each intern's needs.
- Step 3: monthly intern evaluation forms completed by the supervising CML. Ongoing dialogue between supervisors and interns makes the experience more meaningful for both parties.[17] The feedback forms are intended to elicit specific instances of success or areas of improvement and are designed to keep both the supervisor and intern engaged in the experience throughout the course of the internship.

The end goal for this evaluation system is be able to demonstrate value in three ways: to the individual intern, to the institution, and to the profession.

FUTURE DIRECTIONS

Library and college administration consider the WCM/NYP clinical medical library internship program to be a success, and with their support, we plan to continue to recruit for the program and to improve it with each iteration. A Master's degree in library science is simply the first building block for a career in health librarianship. In the absence of formalized CML training programs, internships like this are well positioned to assist librarians in developing necessary skills be successful in CML roles. We suggest other health sciences libraries consider creating their own CML internship program. Interns who experience meaningful, real-world work see the value of the librarian's role and may generate motivation and interest in the field among their peers. By taking this responsibility into our own hands, we can help ensure highly qualified CMLs are ready to fill positions in our own libraries and those across the country.

NOTES

1. B. Baltich Nelson, "Navigating a Path toward a Career in Medical Librarianship," in *Medical Library Association: Librarians Without Borders* (Austin, TX: Medical Library Association, 2015).

2. K. Cimpl, "Clinical Medical Librarianship: A Review of the Literature," *Bull Med Libr Assoc* 73, no. 1 (1985).

3. J. Harrison and V. Beraquet, "Clinical Librarians, a New Tribe in the UK: Roles and Responsibilities," *Health Info Libr J* 27, no. 2 (2010).

4. T. Petrinic and C. Urquhart, "The Education and Training Needs of Health Librarians—the Generalist Versus Specialist Dilemma," *Health Info Libr J* 24, no. 3 (2007).

5. N. B. Giuse et al., "Clinical Medical Librarianship: The Vanderbilt Experience," *Bull Med Libr Assoc* 86, no. 3 (1998).

6. J. A. Lyon et al., "The Lived Experience and Training Needs of Librarians Serving at the Clinical Point-of-Care," *Med Ref Serv Q* 34, no. 3 (2015).

7. B. R. Hendrix and A. E. McKeal, "Case Study: Online Continuing Education for New Librarians," *J Library & Information Services in Distance Learning* 11, nos. 3–4 (2017).

8. D. R. Hill and H. N. Stickell, "Brandon/Hill Selected List of Print Books and Journals for the Small Medical Library," *Bull Med Libr Assoc* 89, no. 2 (2001).

9. L. Kelly and N. St Pierre-Hansen, "So Many Databases, Such Little Clarity: Searching the Literature for the Topic Aboriginal," *Can Fam Physician* 54, no. 11 (2008).

10. S. L. De Groote, M. Shultz, and D. D. Blecic, "Information-Seeking Behavior and the Use of Online Resources: A Snapshot of Current Health Sciences Faculty," *J Med Libr Assoc* 102, no. 3 (2014).

11. I. J. Benjamin et al., *Andreoli and Carpenter's Cecil Essentials of Medicine* (Philadelphia: Elsevier/Saunders, 2016).

12. J. Larry Jameson et al., *Harrison's Principles of Internal Medicine* (New York; Chicago; San Francisco: McGraw Hill Education, 2018).

13. G. B. Green, University Washington, and Department of Medicine, *The Washington Manual of Medical Therapeutics* ([Philadelphia]: Lippincott Williams & Wilkins, 2005).

14. "Request a Systematic Review," Samuel J. Wood Library, https://library.weill.cornell.edu/research-support/research-services/request-systematic-review.

15. J. Brewer and M. D. Winston, "Program Evaluation for Internship/Residency Programs in Academic and Research Libraries," *College & Research Libraries* 62, no. 4 (2001).

16. C. A. Olney et al., *Collecting and Analyzing Evaluation Data* (Seattle, WA; Bethesda, MD: National Network of Libraries of Medicine, Outreach Evaluation Resource Center; National Library of Medicine, 2013).

17. M. Lee, "Growing Librarians: Mentorship in an Academic Library," *Library Leadership & Management* 23, no. 1 (2009).

Chapter Eleven

Making a Clinical Library Service Transformational

Terrie R. Wheeler

This book covered numerous aspects of what a clinical medical librarian (CML) does in various settings or serving specific user groups. Yet several questions remain. How do you build a CML program? How do you make it sustainable? What are the barriers to success, and how are they overcome? What does success look like? Will a value proposition statement help? This chapter intends to answer these questions and more by considering strategic planning, building capacity, developing high-performance teams, and sustaining and assessing programs through the lens of a logic model structured on John Kotter's eight steps for leading change.[1] Kotter's model addresses changing values over time and with recognition that value propositions from one era may not be relevant later. Having developed, renewed, and expanded several CML programs over the years, this author recognized that context and user/stakeholder perceptions of value propositions are key. In the next eight sections, these steps are discussed.

CREATE A SENSE OF URGENCY

Most human beings will not change without an urgent reason. In order to keep a CML program dynamic and forward thinking, one first must create a sense of urgency around the program. This is not difficult. Most CML programs deliver life-altering information when used wisely by clinicians and providers and significantly impact patient care. When starting or breathing new life into a program, a new direction and a new focus of resources are critical to its future success. Identifying or developing clinical champions is a first critical step. Spend time listening to those potential champions. What are the pain points with their current research? Is there an information solution the CML program can offer to address them? Is there a research component of value to the potential champion? Perhaps the value proposition for the potential clinical champion is identifying patients to enroll in the champion's latest clinical trial. The CML can do this by searching de-identified clinical records for patients that match the protocol criteria. In one instance, a CML identified in advance that patients sought for proposed research would be difficult if not impossible to recruit because of the rare combination of study criteria. The researcher valued this information because the CML saved thousands of hours of work.

Listening to clinicians and offering them assistance of marked value can turn them into true CML program champions. Listening to pain points and research program goals is the most effective way to cultivate a potential clinical champion, but it is also critical to keep one's promises and promptly deliver results. This may sound simplistic, and perhaps not even worth mentioning, but reliability cultivates trust and respect. One can build relationship and trust by under-promising and over-delivering. This is a very effective way to continually "wow" a client, and earn the respect and trust necessary to turn that person into a library champion. Many clinical champions are needed to build an effective program. If you have only one or two clinical champions in your entire organization, your program may be considered too parochial, especially by those who are not impacted by its reach.

Once you have won key stakeholders as clinical champions, expand the services you provide them. Can you take the information given at morning report about a very rare case and help the providers develop a case report using articles you provided for discussion? Is a particular case a research interest of one of the providers, and can you offer more research support in that area? Can you recommend the library's systematic reviews service or the library's data service to help that provider further his or her research? This concept of taking a library user deeper into library services that will suit the user's areas of interest through an earlier established trust creates loyal library users who will recommend library services to colleagues and administration.

Changing health care requires a changing value proposition. A blueprint for designing valuable CML services has been to rely on the Joint Commission[2] to identify areas of value for a health-care organization. After all, every hospital needs to meet Joint Commission standards, and using the CML to help them meet these standards has always been a winning strategy.[3] In the 1980s, the Joint Commission standards aligned with hospital departments and included a chapter on the library. In the 1990s the Joint Commission introduced its "Agenda for Change,"[4] which realigned the standards along organizational functions rather than departments. This led to efforts such as CML involvement in occurrence screening,[5] clinical indicator development,[6] and drug use evaluation development.[7] In the 2000s, the CML assumed roles in patient safety and Institutional Review Boards (IRBs) both as a result of the greater emphasis on patient safety required by Joint Commission standards[8] and in response to two deaths of young, healthy volunteer subjects in a clinical trial in 1999[9] and 2001.[10] The Office of Human Research Protection (OHRP) 2001 report, based on a rigorous investigation into the death of the latter subject,[11] found that the Johns Hopkins IRB and/or the principal investigator "failed to find earlier literature demonstrating risks associated with hexamethonium" as the first of three lapses cited in causing the death of this healthy volunteer.[12]

Librarians saw an opportunity to bring their searching skills to the aid of IRBs across the country and got involved in their institutional IRBs.[13] Similarly, librarians and largely CMLs took on other aspects of patient safety, including aspects of knowledge management by sharing knowledge among the health-care team and developing tools to capture tacit or in-house knowledge in the form of lessons learned, which could support organizational learning.[14] CMLs championed the delivery of information to portable devices through work with PDAs,[15] then later through cell phones[16] and other mobile technology. In this decade, CMLs are getting involved in health literacy efforts[17] and actively working with the health-care team through the EMR and app development. (See chapter 7 of this book.)

CMLs have exhibited a remarkable ability to adapt to changing regulations, Joint Commission standards,[18] and organizational and professional needs over the decades. The regulations, review standards, and, in the case of patient deaths, the news media create a sense of urgency around issues that librarians have skills to support or resolve. A library leader's ability to recognize and communicate this sense of urgency to the organization administration and library staff is critical in order to focus available resources on the challenge at hand and to promote new CML initiatives.

PUT TOGETHER THE GUIDING TEAM

Building capacity for the clinical medical librarian program is critical to sustainability and long-term success. Many CML programs consist of librarians who spend only part of their day offering CML services. This may be sufficient in a small community hospital but is not sustainable in a large teaching hospital. Building CML program capacity requires creating a sense of urgency and identifying the most important skillsets needed to address it. It also requires the ability to envision what the organization will need in the future and hire people with broad skillsets who are adaptable and love to learn new things. The guiding team should include the program director, the clinical champion, the CML, and other librarians with an interest in clinical librarianship.

We have discovered clinical medical librarianship is a highly specialized field, making it difficult to hire skilled CMLs. Hence, we have developed our own training program. We hire highly motivated interns with lots of potential and train them by having them shadow senior CMLs. In this way, the interns build their skillset and learn by doing. A well-chosen guiding team will quickly assess the intern's knowledge deficits and help build domain knowledge in one or more medical specialties so the intern can be more effective.

With so many medical specialties today, it is important that the CML is confident and well versed in the subject areas he or she serves regularly, and professional development support is critical to building this domain knowledge. While the informationist model is traditionally more well known for domain expertise,[19] we found that employing the educational model of an informationist to a CML increases the CML's expertise as well as acceptance by the clinical team.

Another way to build capacity is through high-performance teams. High-performance teams function best in a learning organization where they must be flexible and poised to learn new skills in order to accomplish the performance challenge put in front of them. Similar to Collin's BHAG (big hairy audacious goal), a performance challenge brings meaningful purpose to the team.[20] The performance challenge must have specific goals so the team will know when they have met them, and the team must take a common approach to conquering the performance challenge. High-performance teams share leadership, have a deep level of commitment and trust, are mutually accountable to one another, and are willing to learn new skills in order to meet the performance challenge. They spend a lot of time together and build a culture that enables their endeavor to thrive. They are adept problem solvers and have high interpersonal, technical, or functional skills. High-performance teams are known for being relatively small, usually less than ten members. The CML performance challenge is definitely one that engenders and benefits from high-performance teams. Through a shared set of core values, we have seen this occur at the Samuel J. Wood Library.

DEVELOP THE CHANGE VISION AND STRATEGY

Establishing a vision for the CML program and the library is critical. This allows members of the program to engage actively in carrying the vision forward. At the Samuel J. Wood Library, we used the balanced scorecard to develop our overall vision, mission, and core values. The balanced scorecard,[21] a strategic performance measurement model, translates an organization's mission and value into actions. The balanced scorecard's strategy map component is layered on top of the scorecard and is designed to focus attention and resources on select strategic objectives. The CML program actively engages in this effort and could design its own balanced scorecard cascading up to the entire library's balanced scorecard if desired. The CML program focuses concerted efforts on select strategic objectives and develops initiatives to meet them. Development of a balanced scorecard for any organization begins with a SWOT (strengths, weaknesses, opportunities, and threats) analysis followed by a strategic profile. This is an incredibly important aspect of program development. The strategic profile challenges staff members to identify key areas of their industry, and then rank their own organization against at least three other competitors in the market. Through this exercise, staff members see where their organization is strong and where improvement is needed.

An organization defines strengths that make it a "competitive outlier" to other programs and capitalizes on those strengths. At Weill Cornell Medicine (WCM), a high-performance team, our numerous clinical service points, patient reach, access to the electronic medical record, and intern training program are all areas of strength.

Our mission, vision, and core values, championed by our chief information officer, are to transform the library into a pioneering knowledge center that supports next-generation science, health care, and education. The CML program provides support to clinical care of the organization and education to the residents. We work to advance medicine by providing innovative services and access to information through our core values. Our excellence enables us to deliver quality information within two hours of request for patient care, and our innovation created a collaborative environment for residents. For example, we post all pdfs of articles researched by CNLs following morning report in F1000 Workspace, where residents can make notes or highlight the pdfs as appropriate for each case. These often serve as a springboard to a case report.

Over the past year, through quality customer service, we have been asked to expand the CML program to provide service on morning report to other departments. The CML program is one of our library's great strengths, and we play to our strengths. We set our strategy and organizational needs based on our strengths with an eye for the future. Where is health care going? What changes do we anticipate in the Joint Commission standards, and what does that mean for health care? What new technologies are on the horizon, and how will they affect the practice of medicine?

COMMUNICATE FOR UNDERSTANDING AND BUY-IN

Communication is critical. Effective communication can be very difficult to achieve. The beauty of the balanced scorecard is it provides methods for consistent, simple, strategic, and clear communication. The overlaying strategy map enables easy dissemination of the vision and purpose of a program internally to all library staff and externally to stakeholders in administration, in other departments, or to external donors. The messaging is simple and direct. A strategy map illustrating linkage between individual and team efforts to drive the mission, value, and goals of an organization can be highly motivating.

One example of internal communication is a weekly newsletter that covers different aspects of the balanced scorecard and includes examples of individual library staff carrying out specific work to advance a strategic objective or initiative. Over a series of weeks or months, the newsletter represents a picture of the entire scorecard and is an opportunity to brag about some of the internal processes of the library, such as interlibrary loan or counting statistics, both of which are critical to the optimal functions of the library but can seem unimportant. An external communication might be a spreadsheet of library programs provided to potential donors by a development officer.

EMPOWER OTHERS TO ACT

People often want to take action, but they may not know the best route, or there may be barriers preventing them from acting. Thinking back to the change that CMLs experienced over the last several decades, imagine you are a CML in 1994 who sees the Joint Commission eliminate requirements for hospital libraries. Although the library requirement is removed, there are new standards for information management and organizational improvement. Information management requires an assessment of all hospital staff's information needs. This is a role for the library, but new tools may be needed. You know automated survey generators have begun to be deployed, but you do not know how to use one. You can remove this barrier and grow the library's role under the new standard by learning how to use the software. Other members of your team may have different barriers. Listen to your colleagues. What are their barriers? Work with them to remove or reduce the barriers. Enable workarounds, and encourage colleagues to act on the change vision.

For years, CML morning report coverage for the Department of Medicine at WCM was sporadic and supported by individual clinical librarians when staffing allowed. Based on customer feedback, the library director increased morning report coverage by asking interested librarians to participate in a pilot program that covered morning report daily. By dividing the workload between librarians, the pilot program was a success and justified the hire of an additional CML.

PRODUCE SHORT-TERM WINS

We identified quick wins through the pilot program. These include the uptake in number of questions answered by the librarians during the pilot program, and the deeper engagement with the library by the residents and attendings. We received requests to attend morning reports and rounds for other clinical groups where we highlighted additional CML services. We expanded our existing clinical program in pediatrics. An early and highly visible win in pediatrics was creating a fun consumer health information cart. A discarded book cart transformed into a safari jeep driven by a giraffe, Gerald, was a hit on the floor. Gerald and his jeep help engage young pediatric patients and their parents and introduce a positive image of the librarian as part of the health-care team. A development officer heard about the cart and obtained a donation to purchase coloring books containing health and hospital information for distribution to the pediatric patients. Later the donor grew enamored with the service and endowed the CML program. This donor's support provides additional visibility and funding support for the program.

Demand for the CML service grew, and we were able to build momentum for it. We gathered data on the impact of this program in questions answered and presented the results of this effort to the teaching hospital CEO, who agreed this was very helpful to patient care. We wondered not only about the number of questions answered but also how patient care was impacted by the information the CML provided. Consistent with other studies[22] that seek to identify the impact of information provided or its value in a patient-care setting, we developed a value study for the CML program using the critical incident technique methodology. An online link is sent directly to a clinician at the completion of each reference question or search request. The tool asks users to note if the question was answered, not answered, or partially answered. It further considers how the information might have changed the care provided or if it had a financial impact to either the hospital or the patient. For example, did the information help reduce length of stay, change treatment choice, change medication, affect patient mortality, or save health-care provider time? Our goal was to capture quantitative data to demonstrate impact on patient care by a CML program to hospital leadership in the hope of receiving additional funding. We measured the value of short-term wins to estimate future value of program expansion. Demonstrating value builds momentum among the CML team, other library staff, and clinicians and administrators who interface with the program.

DON'T LET UP

It is human nature to want to bask in the success of the recent wins. Do celebrate. It is important to acknowledge victory! Enjoy it with your team, and get used to the taste of success. Nevertheless, how quickly can you as a team push harder for another win, faster for another success? This is the secret to change: the sustained effort to keep accelerating the wins. One must be relentless and seek to ignite change after change once you have discovered a proven model of success. With the changing pace of health care, this is where a sustainable CML program differentiates itself from an unsustainable one. It is relatively easy to have a few quick wins, but it is much harder to have sustained wins over time. The mature and energized CML team recognizes their contributions to health-care information needs to continue to improve and change as health care changes and plays a long game. It is this type of team that rises to become an exemplary CML program in their region or across the country.

By focusing on continuously developing and improving their service as health care changes, this team earns new customer loyalty with deeper levels of service. Clinicians will see the team continually striving to offer the right information at the right time to the right caregivers. Having earned clinicians' trust, the CML team will begin to request services outside of the patient-care setting. Clinicians will trust the CML team to develop new information solutions. Clinicians will be more open to CML recommendations about other library services.

MAKE IT STICK: CREATE A NEW CULTURE

In order to achieve sustainability, the capacity for continuously improving and striving for even greater successes must become part of the organizational culture. Once a leader achieves many quick wins and develops a cadence or rhythm for exceeding goals, the leader is in a position to create a new normal, which includes higher expectations and more reliable products or services. The leader must set these new expectations and continue to remind the team how far they have come. Focus the increased resources resulting from efficiencies or stemming from delighted customers who find your customized services better meet their needs to deliver more value. Then go back to your customers and again listen to their pain points and information needs. What can the highly motivated team do to address other unmet needs? By leveraging the change culture and creating new services, the reach of the

CML team will expand and become relevant in areas not previously considered. Part of establishing the "new normal" for the changed culture of the CML program is using best practices that identify CML program value.

Identifying the value of a knowledge worker has traditionally been challenging because it is very difficult to measure knowledge conveyed or transformed into new knowledge. In health care, knowledge becomes valuable when it facilitates excellent patient care with the least amount of resources. This may be through saving time, preventing needless tests or procedures, avoiding adverse drug reactions, or shortening length of stay. Some best practices for identifying the value of a CML program include:

1. embedding the CML in one or more clinical or translational teams;
2. establishing a Memo of Understanding between the team served and the information center providing the CML;
3. interviewing the team leader to learn the impact of the CML on advancing the mission or science of the team;
4. integrating information into the workflow of the clinical team;
5. cultivating or championing the team's scholarly output;
6. supporting the educational mission of the team in impactful ways; and
7. developing a standardized survey to identify impact of information provided to a team.

Each of these best practices will be discussed individually with examples.

1. Embedding a CML in a clinical team enables a CML who has appropriate domain expertise to function as another team member. In this manner, the library goes to the clinician, rather than vice versa, and the CML can provide the information as needed to advance the clinical care of the team. Physically embedding a CML into a clinical team is not always required to achieve these results. A CML may be assigned to work with several different clinical teams and rotate among them on a weekly or semi-weekly basis. This still achieves the goal of having the CML become a full team member while allowing them to work with several teams, rather than just one or two.
2. Establishing a Memo of Understanding (MOU) between the client clinical team and the CML program allows the library to customize its services to the clinical team being served. These customized services may be documented in the MOU and help define expectations. An MOU can stipulate that the CML is included in all clinical activities of the team and specify that a CML have a mentor on the team who can advise on continuing education to better equip the CML to work with that particular group. Often the MOU outlines periodic requests for feedback on the service, which can include focus groups, survey re-

sponses, or other means for gathering the end user's perspective of the value of the service. In practice, groups receiving CML services at minimal or no charge are eager to provide the mentoring, inclusion in team activities, and evaluation of the efficacy of the CML program in return for gaining a highly skilled and valuable team member.

3. Interviewing the team leader to learn the impact of the CML on advancing the mission of the patient care team is recommended for valuable feedback. The team leader sees the mission of the team in the larger context of the organization as well as the scientific discipline. The team leader may be best able to articulate the value proposition that the CML brings to the clinical care arena and may have recommendations to further integrate the CML into the patient-care setting.

4. Integrating information into the workflow of the team so such information can be engaged when and where it is most needed, while not disrupting the workflow of the clinician, is a goal of the CML. This can be done electronically or by inserting the CML into the workflow process. More often, it includes both approaches. Increasingly the value of the CML is in outlining the workflows of a clinical care process and identifying how master data can be captured once and reused many times for reporting purposes. This concept of developing systems that capture data once, with APIs that export structured data downstream into other systems, is becoming increasingly valued in medical organizations where data-reporting activities are ever increasing but time, staff, and funding are not.

5. The CML can champion the team's scholarly output by locating evidence-based papers that support a particularly challenging clinical diagnosis or therapy. These papers can be placed in a portal environment, such as Faculty 1000 Workspace, where all team members can be granted access to annotate these papers. The CML could then draft a case report for publication with the chief resident or the attending physician by synthesizing what the literature indicates and what the clinical team found to be most effective for this particular case. A step further in this direction would be the CML taking on the role of the managing editor of the case report, involving more members of the team or, if appropriate, recommending a systematic review of similar cases, and taking the librarian lead on the systematic review team. Some ambitious CMLs have taken on the managing editor role of a special issue of a journal and assisted members of the clinical team in each writing one or more articles for this special issue. Efforts like this can get new scientific knowledge into publication months sooner when there is a librarian champion managing the process.

6. The CML may support the continuing medical education of the team by facilitating journal clubs with readings that grant CME credit, by

using their information savvy to introduce new tools, apps, or devices that save clinician's time or by becoming experts who train team members in particular software workflows employed by the team, such as lab notebooks.

In this section, we discussed methods for gathering data on the impact of the CML program, including interviewing the team leader and interviewing a focus group of team members. In the section titled "Produce Short-Term Wins," the quantitative value study approach was discussed. This is a rich source of data over time that will illustrate the value that the CML brings to the team in terms that leadership understands, and can better illustrate the value proposition that the CML provides to the team.

CML PROGRAM ASSESSMENT AND EVALUATION

It is helpful to conduct a periodic assessment of the CML program to review its sustainability and impact on its users. *Assessment* and *evaluation* are often used interchangeably. For the sake of this discussion, consider *assessment* as an understanding of the state or condition of the program and *evaluation* as passing judgment of some kind on the program. In program evaluation, that judgment is often how valuable the program is to the organization.

Program assessment is the process of objectively understanding the state or condition of a program, usually obtained by observation and measurement. A program assessment may be used to evaluate the program. This evaluation or "judgment" is accomplished by comparing it to similar programs or to a standard or by identifying outcomes that the institution deems valuable. There are many ways to conduct an assessment. The balanced scorecard approach reveals much about a program from the four perspectives of customer/stakeholder, internal processes, learning and growth, and financial or budget.

Another method to develop a construct for objectively assessing a program is known as a logic model.[23] A logic model depicts what a program will accomplish through a series of if-then relationships that if, implemented as intended, lead to certain outcomes. A logic model usually contains five categories: resources, activities, outputs, short- and long-term outcomes, and impact. See figure 11.1 for an illustration of a sample logic model for a clinical medical librarian program. This is a thumbnail look at whether a program is accomplishing its goals. Resources are located in the bracket to the left, and activities, outputs, and outcomes align to see if a program is effectively accomplishing its goals. The sample logic model provides CML program activities, outputs, and outcomes, along with resources that go into the program to ensure its success. The outcomes help determine the value of the program to the organization or its success and impact.

PROMOTION STRATEGIES FOR THE CML PROGRAM

CML programs following the best practices for identifying value introduced in the "Make It Stick" section will most likely receive positive word-of-mouth recognition and may not require much promotion. However, there are simple strategies to ensure the CML program and library or information center is integral to the success of the organization. Try to avoid traditional advertising. Focus on marketing to specific user groups based on identified needs instead. What is the difference between advertising and marketing? Advertising makes users aware of a service, usually through announcements geared to large audiences. Marketing involves identifying potential customers and strategically leading a casual or uninterested user through tiers of service that offer increasing customization based on previously identified user needs. This increases the value of the service to the user to the point

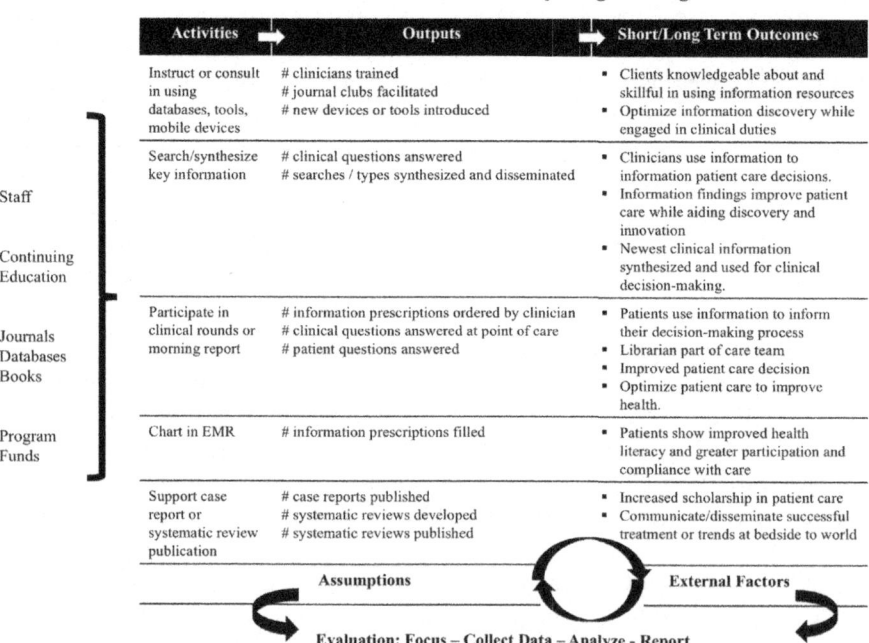

Figure 11.1.   Generic Clinical Medical Library Program Logic Model

where the user becomes a loyal customer and a champion of the company's services to others in the organization.

At an academic organization, you can begin by cultivating the students in their first year. The sooner students, new clinicians, or new investigators become dependent on the services of the information center, the more likely they will return for services that are more complex later. Set up a system of having the team leader or a senior clinician introduce the CML to each new clinician. Include an example of how the CML has supported the clinical care of the senior clinician. In this manner, junior team members will learn the value of and seek out the services offered by the CML.

Develop tiers of customized services from basic to more complex to meet known user needs. See figure 11.2 for an example of tiered services. Introduce new clinicians or investigators to services tailored to their needs. As a new clinician's initial information needs are met, move them along to more advanced services that may exceed their expectations for information services. As expectations are exceeded, and services remain reliable and consistent, the CML cultivates the trust and reliance of the newer clinicians, earning their loyalty over time. This manner of introducing information services is simple, strategic, and highly successful. Once the CML team has developed a series of customized services that meet real needs, the CML team can create a marketing plan that drives users deeper into CML services and promotes customer loyalty to the CML program.

A tier of free introductory services at the top is specifically designed to attract potential customers. A second tier of basic free services delves deeper into what you can offer your customers. A third tier of services is designed to draw the client to increased use of and delight with your services. A fourth tier of services is further customized to individual user needs. The fifth tier consists of the most customizable services you can offer your customers. As clients graduate from one level to the next, they find your services of greater value and, as such, become greater advocates in the organization for your services and your understanding of organizational needs. Those using tier 5 services are likely your most loyal champions.

Following Kotter's eight steps to leading change—using a balanced scorecard, creating high-performance teams, employing best practices, periodically assessing your program, developing a marketing strategy that will demonstrate the value of the program and win loyal program champions—has proven to create sustainable CML programs.

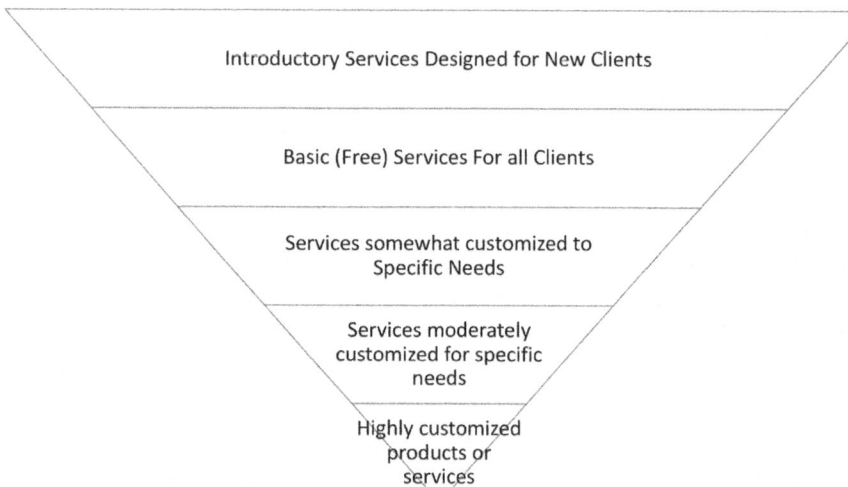

Figure 11.2.   Customer Loyalty Funnel

NOTES

1. John P Kotter, *Leading Change* (Boston: Harvard Business Review Press, 1996).

2. *Joint Commission on Accreditation of Healthcare Organizations* (Oakbrook, IL: The Joint Commission, 2019).

3. P. W. Dalrymple and C. S. Scherrer, "Tools for Improvement: A Systematic Analysis and Guide to Accreditation by the Jcaho," *Bull Med Libr Assoc* 86, no. 1 (1998); J. D. Doyle, "Knowledge-Based Information Management: Implications for Information Services," *Med Ref Serv Q* 13, no. 2 (1994).

4. "Agenda for Change Q&A: Indicators and the Ims (Indicator Monitoring System)," *Jt Comm Perspect* 12, no. 5 (1992); F. Appel, "From Quality Assurance to Quality Improvement: The Joint Commission and the New Quality Paradigm," *J Qual Assur* 13, no. 5 (1991); B. H. Ente, "Stimulating Improved Patient Care: The Joint Commission's Agent for Change," *Top Hosp Pharm Manage* 10, no. 2 (1990).

5. P. B. Howell and C. J. Jones, "A Focus on Quality—the Library's Role in Occurrence Screening," *Med Ref Serv Q* 12, no. 2 (1993).

6. C. Jones, T. Wheeler, and W. Carter, "The Role of Knowledge-Based Information," *SEA Currents* 6, no. 5 (1994).

7. C. B. Good, B. M. Hruska, and T. Wheeler, "Criteria for Long-Term Use of Nonsteroidal Anti-Inflammatory Drugs (Nsaids) in Adult Inpatients and Outpatients," *Clin Pharm* 12, no. 10 (1993).

8. L. Williams and L. Zipperer, "Improving Access to Information: Librarians and Nurses Team up for Patient Safety," *Nurs Econ* 21, no. 4 (2003); L. Zipperer, "Clinicians, Librarians and Patient Safety: Opportunities for Partnership," *Qual Saf Health Care* 13, no. 3 (2004); S. Ramsay, "Johns Hopkins Takes Responsibility for Volunteer's Death," *Lancet* 358, no. 9277 (2001).

9. S. Ramsay, "Johns Hopkins Takes Responsibility for Volunteer's Death," *Lancet* 358, no. 9277 (2001).

10. Ramsay, "Johns Hopkins Takes Responsibility"; Robert Steinbrook, "Protecting Research Subjects—the Crisis at Johns Hopkins," *N Engl J Med* 346, no. 9 (2002).

11. Associated Press, "OHRP Suspends Johns Hopkins Research License for Fed Funded Research," http://ahrp.org/ohrp-suspends-johns-hopkins-research-license-for-fed-funded-research.

12. Donald Kennedy, "Death at Johns Hopkins" (American Association for the Advancement of Science, 2001).

13. Judith G. Robinson and Jessica Lipscomb Gehle, "Medical Research and the Institutional Review Board: The Librarian's Role in Human Subject Testing," *Reference Services Review* 33, no. 1 (2005); Robert V. Labaree, "Working Successfully with Your Institutional Review Board: Practical Advice for Academic Librarians," *College & Research Libraries News* 71, no. 4 (2010), https://crln.acrl.org/index.php/crlnews/article/view/8353/8494.

14. Zipperer, "Clinicians, Librarians and Patient Safety."

15. Jean P. Shipman and Andrew C. Morton, "The New Black Bag: Pdas, Health Care and Library Services," *Reference Services Review* 29, no. 3 (2001); C. Honeybourne, S. Sutton, and L. Ward, "Knowledge in the Palm of Your Hands: Pdas in the Clinical Setting," *Health Info Libr J* 23, no. 1 (2006).

16. S. Krishna, S. A. Boren, and E. A. Balas, "Healthcare Via Cell Phones: A Systematic Review," *Telemed J E Health* 15, no. 3 (2009).

17. Connie Schardt, "Health Information Literacy Meets Evidence-Based Practice," *Journal of the Medical Library Association: JMLA* 99, no. 1 (2011); Nancy D. Zionts et al., "Promoting Consumer Health Literacy," *Reference & User Services Quarterly* 49, no. 4 (2011).

18. *Joint Commission on Accreditation of Healthcare Organizations*; Joint Commission on Accreditation of Healthcare Organizations, *The Measurement Mandate: On the Road to Performance Improvement in Health Care* (Oakbrook Terrace, IL: Joint Commission, 1993).

19. S. F. Grefsheim et al., "The Informationist: Building Evidence for an Emerging Health Profession," *J Med Libr Assoc* 98, no. 2 (2010); J. A. Rankin, S. F. Grefsheim, and C. C. Canto, "The Emerging Informationist Specialty: A Systematic Review of the Literature," *J Med Libr Assoc* 96, no. 3 (2008).

20. James C. Collins and Jerry I. Porras, *Built to Last: Successful Habits of Visionary Companies*, 10th revised ed. (New York: Harper Business, 2004).

21. Robert S. Kaplan et al., *The Strategy-Focused Organization: How Balanced Scorecard Companies Thrive in the New Business Environment* (Boston: Harvard Business Press, 2001).

22. D. N. King, "The Contribution of Hospital Library Information Services to Clinical Care: A Study in Eight Hospitals," *Bull Med Libr Assoc* 75, no. 4 (1987); K. Dunn et al., "Measuring the Value and Impact of Health Sciences Libraries: Planning an Update and Replication of the Rochester Study," *J Med Libr Assoc* 97, no. 4 (2009).

23. Logic Model Development Guide, (Battle Creek, MI: W.K. Kellogg Foundation, 2004), https://greatnetworkglobal.org/resource-library/using-logic-models-to-bring-together-planning-evaluation-and-action.

Index

About the Editor and Contributors

Judy C. Stribling is the assistant director of clinical services at the Samuel J. Wood Library & C.V. Starr Biomedical Information Center at Weill Cornell Medical College. She is also the manager of the Myra Mahon Patient Resource Center or PRC. Judy and other clinical medical librarian team members impact patient care through many activities, including: rounding with providers, attending morning reports, providing targeted evidence-based literature on topics of relevance to current clinical cases, and assisting physicians with the identification and integration of mobile information tools into their clinical workflows. Additionally, Judy teaches medical literature searching skills in the application of evidence-based medicine in the neurology clerkship.

In her role at the PRC, Judy and her staff provide free up-to-date information about diseases, medications, and wellness topics to patients, families, and caregivers. Health consumers are welcome to visit the PRC during scheduled health and wellness seminars, to conduct research on the PRC computers, to relax in between appointments, or to consult with Judy.

Consumer health and the integration of technology and patient education is the focus of Judy's academic interests. Recent research has focused on the introduction of electronic tablets in clinical waiting areas and health seminars on YouTube.

Judy received the Medical Library Association's 2019 Consumer Health Librarian of the Year Award. She is a past chair of the Consumer and Patient Health Information Section (CAPHIS) of the Medical Library Association (MLA). She is also certified by MLA as an Academy of Health Information Professional (AHIP) and Consumer Health Information Specialist.

* * *

Becky Baltich Nelson is a clinical and systems librarian at the Samuel J. Wood Library at Weill Cornell Medicine. In this role, she works with New York Presbyterian Hospital's Department of Medicine and Department of Pediatrics to provide evidence-based literature to clinical teams and consumer health information to patients and their families. Additionally, she is a member of the library's systematic review service and manages the library's Balanced Scorecard. She is a member of the Medical Library Association and works as an internet researcher for a private investigation firm. She holds a B.S. in psychology from the University of Wisconsin–Superior, an M.S. in college counseling and student development from St. Cloud State University, and an M.L.S. from the University of Maryland.

Michelle Demetres is a scholarly communications librarian at the Samuel J. Wood Library, Weill Cornell Medicine, assisting and supporting researchers in all aspects of the scholarly publishing lifecycle. As a member of the WCM faculty, Michelle has developed and taught courses to a range of health professionals and students, helping to incorporate research skills and resources into the curriculum. Michelle is also an active collaborator in the library's systematic review service, grant-editing service, and institutional repository. She holds a B.A. from James Madison University, and a master's of library and information science (MLIS) from Queens College.

As a faculty member of the Samuel J. Wood Library at Weill Cornell Medical College, **Antonio P. DeRosa** serves as the oncology consumer health librarian, which is a patient- and caregiver-oriented clinical role specializing in oncology information, education, and managing patient-focused oncology resources within the Myra Mahon Patient Resource Center. Antonio works in close collaboration with the Oncology Service Line at New York-Presbyterian Hospital and on interdisciplinary teams in the Weill Cornell Medicine Sandra and Edward Meyer Cancer Center. He is an active member of the Medical Library Association (MLA) on national and local levels, and a senior member of the Academy of Health Information Professionals (AHIP). Antonio holds an M.S. in library and information science (MLIS) from Pratt Institute and an M.S. in data science from Elmhurst College. His research interests include health literacy, participatory medicine, patient-centered care, and informed decision support.

As a research informationist III, **Marisol Hernandez** was part of the reference team at the Memorial Sloan Kettering Cancer Center Library. Serving as the embedded clinical librarian liaison to the nursing department, Marisol collaborated with nursing staff at all levels on evidence-based practice (EBP) projects, as well as lecture and teaching assignments, and participated in various nursing councils such as nursing practice, nursing informatics, and nursing research. Most importantly, she participated in the cancer center's journey to Magnet Status, resulting in Magnet achievement in 2016. Additionally, she has expertise in conducting systematic reviews with interdisciplinary clinical and research teams. Ms. Hernandez is a faculty member with the City College of New York (CCNY)/CUNY School of Medicine (CSOM) serving as an associate professor-medical librarian.

Her educational attainments include bachelor of arts in music from Hobart and William Smith Colleges; master of arts in American studies and master of library science from the State University of New York at Buffalo; and certificate in health-care informatics from Drexel University.

Keith C. Mages is a clinical medical librarian at the Samuel J. Wood Library of Weill Cornell Medicine, where he provides research and evidence-based practice support to practicing physicians, nurses, medical fellows, residents, and students. He holds a B.S. in nursing and an M.L.S. from the University at Buffalo, as well as a master's in child and adolescent psychiatric nursing (MSN) from Yale University and a Ph.D. in the history of nursing from the University of Pennsylvania. He is a senior member of the Medical Library Association's Academy of Health Information Professionals with research interests in health literacy, patient education, and the history of health care.

Loretta Merlo is a thirty-eight-year veteran of the Samuel J. Wood Library at Weill Cornell. Thirty-five of those years have been spent in the public service area as manager of circulation services, where she interacts with library patrons, especially medical students, every day. Since its inception in 2006, Loretta has been the architect of the Library Treasure Hunt, an idea originally proposed by Helen-Ann Brown, MLS.

Dr. Nena Osorio is vice chair for quality and patient safety and associate professor of clinical pediatrics in the Department of Pediatrics, Weill Cornell Medicine. She is also associate attending at New York-Presbyterian Hospital/Weill Cornell Medical Center and the NYP Komansky Children's Hospital.

Dr. Osorio received her medical degree from the University of Belgrade School Of Medicine in 1985. From 1987 to 1992, Dr. Osorio conducted basic science research as a visiting fellow and postdoctoral associate in the Department of Physiology and Biophysics at Cornell Medical College. During this period, her work resulted in three publications in peer-reviewed journals. Dr. Osorio completed pediatric residency training in 1995, and she served as a chief resident in 1996. She was a practicing pediatrician until 2003, at which point she returned to Weill Cornell Medical College (WCMC) and New York-Presbyterian Hospital/Weill Cornell Medical Center as the medical director for the General Pediatric Inpatient Unit. She served as medical director until June 2017. Dr. Osorio assumed a new role as a director of quality, patient safety, and family engagement in July 2017, leading departmental efforts at improving patient safety and quality. In March 2018, Dr. Osorio was appointed as vice chair of quality and patient safety in the Department of Pediatrics.

In 2011, Dr. Osorio obtained a master's in translational and clinical research and completed a fellowship in health care quality and medical informatics. In 2017, she completed the Advanced Improvement Methods at Cincinnati Children's Hospital, which focused on advanced quality improvement techniques. Dr. Osorio's main research interests are in improving safe transitions from hospital to home and thereby improving clinical care. She authored and co-authored over sixteen manuscripts that were published in peer-reviewed journals. She is the site PI for the American Academy of Pediatrics QI collaborative "Improving Pediatric Patient-Centered Transitions," which designed and implemented pediatric discharge bundle, resulting in a manuscript in *Pediatrics, 2016*. This research confirmed that patients with complex medical needs, particularly those who are technology-supported (with tracheostomy tubes, feeding tubes, central lines, and VP shunts), have high health-care utilization and need special attention in transitions from hospital to home. Dr. Osorio helped develop a clinical program known as "The Simulation-Based Discharge Program," which provides training to enable the caregivers of patients with newly placed devices to care for them at home. This program consists of two components, namely, Simulation-Based Patient Education (SBPE) and support provided by parent volunteers (Parent-to-Parent support team—P-2-P) to improve comfort, knowledge, and skills for caregivers in managing children's new medical devices outside the hospital. The P-2-P support team is comprised of parents whose children had or still have tracheostomy tubes. This team represents a subgroup of parents who belong to the Family Advisory Council (FAC). This program received the International Patient and Family Centered Care Award as an exemplary, innovative partnership between medical staff and parents/caregivers in December 2017. This program allows patients to transition directly from hospital to home, bypassing the need for chronic care facility stays and holding promise to reduce thirty-day readmissions (research in progress). In her new role, Dr. Osorio serves as the local and regional leader for the Solution for Patient Safety (SPS).

Robert P. Oxley is the associate director of research services at the Samuel J. Wood Library & C.V. Starr Biomedical Information Center. In this capacity, he oversees provisioning and education in research applications, databases, and services. This includes managing the institutional Data Core, a secure enclave cloud computing environment for storage and analysis of clinical data; establishing the library bioinformatics service; teaching and consulting in data science and bioinformatics; and managing the Scientific Software Hub for discovery and provisioning of software licensing across the institution. His research interests include data literacy, scientific reproducibility, machine learning, and bioinformatics. Peter has a Ph.D. in behavioral genetics and evolution from the University of Sydney, a graduate diploma in genetic counseling from Newcastle University, and a bachelor's in molecular biology and genetics (with honors) from the University of Sydney.

Rachel Pinotti is the associate library director for education and research services at the Icahn School of Medicine at Mount Sinai (ISMMS). In this role, she serves as co-director of the longitudinal evidence-based medicine (EBM) curriculum, working with medical education administration and faculty to ensure that EBM is included in the curriculum in a robust and meaningful way. Rachel serves as course director for the Introduction to Systematic Reviews course and co-course director for the Lessons in Scientific Publishing course in the Graduate School of Biomedical Sciences. Rachel also oversees reference, consultation, and instruction services for ISMMS and the hospitals of the Mount Sinai Health System. She enjoys working with a diverse group of patrons including medical and graduate students, faculty, residents, fellows, and staff.

Rachel earned her B.A. summa cum laude from Emory University and her master of science in library and information science (MLIS) from the Palmer School of Library and Information Science. She is a senior member of the Academy of Health Information Professionals (AHIP).

Timothy Roberts, MLS, MPH, is a medical librarian with over twenty years' experience in a variety of health sciences libraries and the information solutions industry. He is currently the population health librarian/associate curator at the NYU Health Sciences Library, NYU School of Medicine. In this role, he supports the Department of Population Health by collaborating on systematic reviews, instructing new faculty and staff in effective literature searching, and providing support in information discovery from nontraditional resources.

Tim has worked as a medical librarian in a variety of health sciences libraries, including the National Network of Libraries of Medicine, the New York Academy of Medicine, and the Michael Callen—Audre Lorde Community Health Center and the Hospital for Special Surgery. He spent five years at Ovid Technologies, both licensing health information content and specifying technical requirements for the development of new products and enhancement of the existing search platform. He has also developed and taught the master's-level course Information Retrieval and Virtual Libraries for the

SUNY Downstate Medical Center, College of Health Related Professions, Medical Informatics Program.

Tim holds a master's of library science (MLS) from the University at Buffalo, the State University of New York, and a master's of public health from CUNY School of Public Health at Hunter College.

Terrie R. Wheeler was appointed the director of the Samuel J. Wood Library and C.V. Starr Biomedical Information Center in 2014 to lead a library transformation to a facility supporting next-generation science, care, and education at Weill Cornell Medicine. She has over thirty-five years of experience in medical librarianship that enables her to effectively lead change. Early in her career, she introduced clinical medical library services in hospital or health-care institutions where she worked. At Weill Cornell, she has championed the dramatic expansion of these services, and sought to ensure librarians had access to the electronic health record, as they are such integral members of the multidisciplinary care team.

She believes that patients get better care when they, their families, and their clinical care team receive health information in a timely manner from trained clinical medical librarians.

She has held supervisory positions since 1991 at the Department of Veterans Affairs, the National Institutes of Standards and Technology, the Walter Reed Army Institute of Research, and the National Institutes of Health Library. Terrie holds bachelor's degrees in biology and English from Adrian College, and a master's in library science from the University of Michigan.

Michael Wood serves as the head of resource management at the Samuel J. Wood Library of Weill Cornell Medicine. In this role, he coordinates and manages all aspects of the library's collection development and technical services activities, including acquisitions, cataloging, serials, e-resources, EZproxy, and so on. Michael holds a B.S. and M.L.S. from the City University of New York's City College and Queens College, respectively.

Drew Wright is the scholarly communications librarian at Weill Cornell Medical Library, where he serves as a liaison between the library and the research community and provides support to students and faculty regarding publishing, government policy, experimental design, and data management. Drew has a bachelor's degree in chemical engineering and a master's in library and information science.

Made in the USA
Coppell, TX
16 June 2023

18163391R00100